BASIC FITNESS

Also by the author:
Basic Judo
In preparation:
Basic Karate

BASIC FITNESS

E. G. Bartlett

DAVID & CHARLES
NEWTON ABBOT LONDON
NORTH POMFRET (VT) VANCOUVER

ISBN 0 7153 7172 X
Library of Congress Catalog Card Number 76-1402

Set in 11pt on 13pt Times New Roman
by Trade Linotype Limited, Birmingham
and printed in Great Britain
by Redwood Burn Ltd, Trowbridge and Esher

for David & Charles (Publishers) Limited
Brunel House Newton Abbot Devon

Published in the United States of America
by David & Charles Inc
North Pomfret Vermont 05053 USA

Published in Canada
by Douglas David & Charles Limited
1875 Welch Street North Vancouver BC

Contents

Introduction

It is not so many years ago that fitness was the preoccupation of the health and strength enthusiast, the body-builder, or the hypochondriac. Today, however, millions of ordinary people are realising that it concerns them. The quality of our lives is bound up with physical fitness. In this book, we shall look at those factors which make us fit; we shall identify the dangers to good health; we shall learn the cures. In learning how our bodies work and what they need to function efficiently, we shall understand what we can do to help ourselves.

Fitness is based on correct eating habits and regular exercise. For the average person, this does not mean drastic dieting or rigorous training. It means simply seeing that we eat the right foods in the right quantities to supply our body's needs, and that we get enough exercise to keep our bodies in trim.

The main dangers to fitness today arise from our sedentary occupations and pastimes, from our processed foods, from the stresses of modern life – particularly city life – and from lack of fresh air. The killer diseases today are not consumption or pneumonia: new drugs and better living standards have helped us to cope with those. The killer diseases today are coronary failures, fatty degeneration of the heart, thrombosis, ulcers and obesity. They are the ills of affluence.

Our social habits are partly to blame for these diseases. Too many city workers spend all day seated at an office desk and then go home to sit in front of the television all evening. Many factory workers are often exercising only a small number of muscles in some highly repetitive movement on a conveyor belt. Usually even these movements are performed sitting still in one spot. The number of people who could be considered to get enough exercise for health from their daily occupation is diminishing, and every new labour-saving device and modern aid makes the position worse. Automation has many blessings; it takes over so much of the work that was once pure drudgery, but pushing a button does not provide the same exercise as wielding a hammer, nor using a vacuum cleaner the same exercise as beating a carpet; and unused muscles have a tendency to atrophy.

Exercise helps us in three ways: it preserves our muscles in a usable condition; it improves our breathing and circulation; it increases our metabolism, so enabling us to digest our food more readily.

Lack of exercise weakens our muscles, causes deterioration in our breathing and circulation, and slows down our metabolism. The significance of a lower metabolic rate is that if our food intake is constant, not all of it is used up before the next intake and so we grow fat, with all the dangers to health and happiness that that entails.

A diet of entirely fresh food has probably not been known since men lived in caves and hunted with bow and arrow. It was learned quite early in man's history that food starts to deteriorate as soon as it is gathered, whether it be crops from the fields or meat from the slaughter-house. Men have found ways of arresting this deterioration. The usual methods of preserving food are drying, refrigeration, canning, dehydration and preserving by additives. Drying and refrigeration have been in use for centuries, even before the refrigerator as we know it was even thought of. Canning, dehydration and the use of additives are more modern methods.

Today many housewives are out at work, and it is clearly easier for them to open a tin of peas than to shell and cook them. The demand for preserved foods has therefore increased. We need to look at the dangers of these preserved and processed foods, but we need to do so without alarmist preconceptions.

The main nutrients affected by food processing are vitamins B_1 and C. Quick-freezing of vegetables will cause very little loss of vitamin C, but leaving them to dry on the plant before canning them will produce a very great loss. Frozen vegetables, therefore, are generally to be preferred to canned ones.

Food that is going to be canned is sterilised by heating. Meats need to be heated to a higher temperature than vegetables and vegetables to a higher temperature than fruits, so that the loss of vitamin B_1 in meat may be as high as 60–70 per cent. Sometimes the manufacturer replaces these losses by adding vitamins to the finished product; sometimes he does not. Unless the manufacturer has replaced vitamins, therefore, canned meats will have lost more vitamins than vegetables or fruits. We need to study carefully the labels on tins.

There is government control over the colouring and other additives that can be used in foods, so that the public is generally well protected in that respect.

Our love of white bread means that the loaf we

eat is deficient in nutritional value, despite the enrichment of which some manufacturers boast. The most important item missing from the white loaf is fibre, which is valuable to the human body as a laxative. We can get this fibre by eating wholemeal bread, but this is generally more expensive than white bread and sometimes not as easy to obtain.

Some people live on 'natural foods', that is on those grown on soil that is fertilised by organic fertilisers. Some people eschew meat and poultry produced by factory farming methods, either on humanitarian grounds or because they do not believe that the product is as good. We must concede that health foods have many advantages. They are more natural for they have not lost vitamins or roughage. On the other hand they do tend to be more expensive than those normally available in the supermarket. Although the people who live solely on natural foods are undoubtedly healthy, this is not of itself conclusive evidence that those foods are more nutritious, since such people usually take many other precautions to safeguard their health as well, and these other factors must be taken into account when assessing the end result.

In general, we must accept that processed foods are here to stay, and that because they are cheaper they will inevitably form part of the daily diet for most families. If there is a choice available, by all means let us prefer natural foods, but if not, let us by attention to our diet see that our processed foods are giving us adequate quantities of the various elements we need to keep us fit.

We have spoken earlier of the stresses of modern living. The pace of city life, the noise, the air pollution, the personal conflicts of the rat race, anxieties over our future, all these things affect us. It is only a very few who can, or who want, to opt out. For most of us it is a case of learning to live with stress.

To do this we must adopt the right attitudes. Some things we can change; some we cannot. We need the wisdom to separate the one from the other, and the resignation to accept cheerfully what cannot be altered.

It may help to realise that anger does far more harm to us than to the person or circumstance that makes us angry. Impatience over trivialities can only raise our blood pressure; it cannot put things right. For most of us calmness and inner serenity are ideals, but they are ideals at which to aim, and which, if achieved, will benefit our health. 'Let not the sun go down upon your wrath' is not only sound religious doctrine, it is good advice from the health point of view.

The dangers of smoking have received so much publicity that it is hardly necessary to restate them. The dangers of overindulgence in alcohol are likewise well known. Moderation in all things is the rule of health.

'Early to bed and early to rise makes a man healthy, wealthy and wise' is an old country saying, and it is perfectly true. One hour in bed before midnight is worth two after. In the adult needs vary as to sleep, but eight hours work, eight hours leisure and eight hours sleep is a fair division of a man's day.

To sum up, the general rules for healthy living are:

1 Eat the right foods in the right quantities.

2 Get sufficient daily exercise to keep all your muscles in trim.

3 Adopt a calm, serene attitude to life.

4 Avoid excess in drinking. Give up smoking. Avoid drugs.

5 Live moderately and simply.

6 If you are still not satisfied with your standard of fitness, decide now to do something about it. This book will tell you how.

1
Nutritional Needs for Health and Fitness

We are what we eat. That is the truth in its simplest form. Apart from oxygen and water, which is itself a part of our food, all the physical components of our bodies are made of food. Initially our bodies are built up from food derived from our mother. Then they are developed by the food we eat during childhood and adolescence. Finally, when we have reached maturity, they are maintained by the food we eat throughout our adult lives.

The human body is like a machine that does its own running repairs. As cells wear out or break down, so they are replaced or repaired. Every single cell in our body is replaced over a period of seven years.

Food is therefore essential for three reasons: because it provides the raw materials for growth and later for replacements and repairs; because it provides energy for carrying out our bodily functions, and by these we mean not only our conscious movements, but also the involuntary actions of our glands, nervous systems and organs, which go on even when we are asleep; because it provides energy for warmth.

If we are deprived of the food we need when we are growing, we shall not become strong, healthy adults. If we are deprived after we have reached maturity, the replacement and repair service will break down and we will fall ill or age prematurely.

But it is not just any food that we require; it is the right food in the right quantities. In this chapter we shall consider our nutritional requirements more deeply and learn what we need and where we get those needs supplied. Basically our requirements can be divided into seven groups: proteins, carbohydrates, fats, minerals, vitamins, roughage and other elements. Let us consider each group in turn.

PROTEINS

Our bodies, like those of every living creature, are made up of countless cells. We begin life in our mother's womb as two cells, the ova being fertilised by the spermatozoa. Cells then rapidly multiply, and our cells divide and become parts of specialised organs such as the heart, the liver, the lungs and the skin, all of which have their own function to perform in keeping us alive. The cells of all these organs are made of proteins.

Proteins are chemical compounds of carbon, oxygen, hydrogen and nitrogen, combined with other elements such as phosphorus and sulphur. Protein molecules are built up of amino acids, and when we eat protein it is broken down in our stomachs and intestines into its constituent amino acids, which are then absorbed into the capillaries of the small intestine and used for the growth, repair or replacement of cells. The body has the ability to combine the amino acids according to different formulae so as to create the various kinds of protein needed to build up different cells. Thus some will be converted into blood cells, others into muscle cells, etc. The raw materials are carried in the blood stream to the particular part of the body where they are needed.

Protein is mainly to be found in foods derived from animals, both directly, as in meat or fish, and indirectly, as in eggs or milk. It can also be found in plants, again directly, as in peas and beans, or indirectly, as in bread. Because the animal proteins are very similar to our own, they will of themselves provide all the amino acids we need. If we rely on the vegetable ones, however, some plants may be deficient in certain proteins, and this must be overcome by mixing our vegetables so that what is lacking in one can be found in another. It is quite possible to do this, of course, and what has been said is no argument against a strictly vegetarian diet, but the best way to obtain our protein requirements, as well as the cheapest, is to combine meat and vegetables on our plate. This is reflected in our traditional English dishes such as roast beef with vegetables, or fish with peas and chips.

The quantities of protein we need vary with our age and the kind of life we lead, and to some extent with our sex also, women needing slightly less than men. Obviously a very active man such as a heavy manual labourer or a weight-lifter training for a competition is going to break down more cells in a day than an office worker who goes home and sits by the fireside all the evening.

As a guide, we say that infants at 2 years need 30g of protein per day. This rises steadily until at 9 years they need 55g per day. An 18-year-old boy needs 75g per day; an 18-year-old girl, 58g per day. From that age onwards the daily requirement of the female is 12 or 13g less than the male. An active young man will need 90g per day, a moderately active one 75, and one pursuing a purely sedentary life may manage with 70. These figures will decrease again as old age approaches and may come down to 55g again. During pregnancy and while breast feeding, a woman's need increases, so that at these times 10g per day could be added to the above figures. These are broad guidelines. Our body is adapted to dealing with excess; if we take in too much, it is simply eliminated. It is only if we take too little that trouble will arise.

To talk of so many grammes of protein, however, may not mean very much to the ordinary man or woman. How many of us can visualise what a gramme would look like? Protein is only a part of any particular serving of food, and 100g of meat do not contain 100g of protein or anything like that quantity. It will be helpful therefore if we have some guide as to what a particular item on our plate might be expected to contain.

Meat contains about 7g per ounce, so a 6oz (170g) steak contains 42g. Cheese is the same value as meat; fish 6g per ounce; bread and other foods made of grain $2\frac{1}{2}$g per ounce; beans, peas and similar vegetables 2g per ounce; one egg contains 7g.

We can see, therefore, that it is only a case of simple arithmetic to make sure we get our basic requirement, and it is a fact that normal, well-balanced family meals do provide our needs providing they are sufficiently varied.

CARBOHYDRATES

Carbohydrates, together with fats, give us energy. The unit of energy is the calorie, which in this sense is not the calorie we speak of in physics, but 1,000 times as great. Strictly speaking our calorie should be spelt with a capital C, but it is not usually done in textbooks on nutrition, so we will omit doing so also. The main thing we have to bear in mind when assessing our calorie requirements is that those calories which are not burnt up as energy are stored as fat, so we must not take in more than we need.

There are three main groups of carbohydrates:

1 Monosaccharides. These are simple sugars.

2 Disaccharides. These are made up of two simple sugar molecules.

3 Polysaccharides. These are complex groups such as starches.

Carbohydrates can only be absorbed by the body in their simplest form as monosaccharides, so that the more complex forms have to be broken down by the digestive processes. They are then absorbed into the blood stream which carries them to the part of the body where they are needed.

The amount of sugar in the blood stream is known as the blood sugar level. Some of the sugar is removed by a hormone called insulin and is stored. When the blood sugar level drops, as it will do an hour or so after a meal, some of the reserves of sugar that have been stored will be called upon. A drop in blood sugar level is thought to be one of the causes of our feeling hungry.

We get carbohydrates from all sugars and starches. The commonest source is sugar itself, but supplies also come from fruit, honey, flour, bread, cereals, potatoes, rice, semolina, lentils and beans.

The quantities we need must be taken in conjunction with fats. About 50 per cent of our energy is provided by our carbohydrate intake, 35–40 per cent by fats, and the remainder from protein foods. Once again, how many calories we need per day from all sources depends on age, sex and the degree of our activity.

Infants at 2 need 1,200 calories per day, rising to 2,100 at 9. At 18, a boy needs 3,000 and a girl 2,300. An active man will need 3,600, a moderately active one 3,000 and a sedentary worker 2,700. A very active woman needs 2,500 but the normal is 2,200, apart from times of pregnancy or breast feeding when from 200 to 500 can be added. These figures all decrease in men and women with the onset of old age and drop back to just over 2,000 per day, assuming of course a less active life.

Consider that 50 per cent of these calories are coming from carbohydrates. Again 'gram of carbohydrate' is rather a meaningless term to most of us. What we need is something we can visualise on our plate. An average helping of cereal would contain 20g; so would a slice of bread, 4oz (113g) of butter beans, lentils or peas; a large apple would contain 12g. We need not worry unduly if the number of calories we get from carbohydrates is low, providing it is supplemented with calories from protein or fat. Protein must always be considered a better source of calories than carbohydrates, particularly if we want to keep slim.

FATS

Fats are another source of calories, as we have just said, and they are twice as rich in calories as carbohydrates. Fats do much more than give us some of our calories, however. They assist growth and development, they insulate the body against cold, and they make our food more palatable. Consider bread without butter, and you will understand what fats do for food.

We get fats from the obvious sources such as butter, lard, dripping, meat, olive oil and margarine, and also from less obvious sources such as fish and eggs. Our daily need must be calculated with our total calorie need.

MINERALS

Minerals help the growth and repair of the body. Our main mineral requirements are calcium and iron. Calcium is needed to build and maintain our bones and teeth and to help our blood to clot if we cut ourselves. Iron is essential to the red corpuscles of the blood, and deficiency leads to anaemia. Another mineral we must have is phosphorus, which is used in the chemical reactions that turn our food into energy.

Apart from these main minerals, there are many others that are required in minute quantities, and these are called 'trace elements'. Trace elements are defined as those that are one part in twenty thousand of the organism. Of these trace elements, copper combines with iron to make haemoglobin, cobalt is used in the manufacture of red blood cells in bone marrow, zinc becomes part of an enzyme concerned with tissue respiration, manganese helps to release energy from food, iodine helps the metabolic process and the thyroid gland, fluorine is needed for bone tissue, for preventing dental decay and for the thyroid gland and the skin, and salts are needed to regulate the concentration of body fluid.

Where do we get these minerals? Calcium comes from milk, cheese, cereals and bread; iron from liver, kidneys and hearts especially, but also from cereals, green vegetables and eggs; phosphorus, in the minute quantities that we need it, is found in most foods but especially in liver, kidneys, beef, mutton, cheese, eggs, wholemeal bread and milk. The trace elements are found in any diet that includes meat, vegetables and fish as well as dairy products.

Our daily needs of calcium and iron are large enough to be measured and are as follows:

Calcium

Up to 9 years – 500mg per day.
9–15 years – 700mg per day.

18 years – 600mg per day (a decrease with a steady decrease thereafter to 500mg per day).

This need is the same for men and women, except that during pregnancy a woman's need will increase to 1,200mg per day.

Iron

Up to 3 years – 7mg per day.

4–7 years – 8mg per day.

7–9 years – 10mg per day.

18 years – 15mg per day.

Needs then level off at the decreased level of 12mg per day for both men and women, except during pregnancy when a woman's need will be 15mg per day.

VITAMINS

Vitamins are substances which are required in very small quatities for the maintenance of health. They are quite distinct from carbohydrates, fats, proteins and mineral salts. Their absence from our diet leads to deficiency diseases, a fact which was known long before the term 'vitamin' was first used in the 1920s. Thus for centuries sailors knew that they needed fresh fruit to prevent scurvy.

There are about twenty-seven identified vitamins at the moment. Seven of them are known to be essential to us and the rest are presumed to be.

Vitamin A is needed to keep the skin and the breathing passages healthy. It is found in cod-liver oil, halibut oil, the liver of animals, eggs, butter and milk. Our daily requirement is 5,000iu.

Vitamin B is not a single vitamin but a group known as the 'vitamin B complex'. B_1 is needed to prevent such diseases as beri-beri and neuritis. It is found in brewer's yeast, wheat germ, peas, haricot beans, egg yolk and wholemeal flour. Men need 1–5mg per day; women between 1 and 2mg. B_2 consists of a number of substances usually known by their chemical names. Riboflavin feeds the body cells, and its absence causes skin and eye troubles. It is found in yeast, milk, eggs, fish roes and liver. Men need 1–6mg per day; women 1–4mg. Nicotinic acid prevents pellagra and helps to combat tuberculosis. It is found in yeast, liver, fish, meat and wholemeal flour. A man needs 15mg per day; a woman 12mg. Folic acid and vitamin B_{12} help in the formation of blood. Folic acid is found in liver and green vegetables, and B_{12} in liver, yeast, cereals and pulses. The daily requirement is unknown.

Vitamin C is needed to build healthy tissue and to aid the metabolism of individual cells. If it is lacking, wounds do not heal, bones and teeth are abnormal and haemorrhages may occur. Men need 75mg per day; women 70mg. The best sources are fresh fruit and green vegetables, particularly blackcurrants, oranges, lemons, strawberries, apples and cabbage.

Vitamin D aids the digestion of calcium, so that its absence leads to deformities of the bones or teeth. It is found in fish, cod-liver oil and halibut-liver oil, but is also obtained from sunlight falling on the skin, which makes sunbathing so desirable an activity. Men and women need from 400 to 800iu per day.

Vitamin E has been found necessary for the functioning of the reproductive system in animals. Normally this is found so readily in a man's diet that there has been no proper study of deficiency in the human being, so evidence is lacking to show whether such deficiency might affect sexual performance. It is found in wheat germ and rice germ, oils, cotton-seed oil, lettuce and spinach and in eggs. The daily requirement is not known.

Vitamin K is needed to make the blood clot. It is found in spinach, spring greens and in dark green vegetables. Vitamin P is called 'citrin'. It is needed to make the capillaries strong, and to help with the formation of red blood cells and the production of antibodies. Lack of this vitamin leads to capillary haemorrhages. It is found in blackcurrants, oranges, lemons, rosehips and green vegetables. Very minute quantities of both vitamin K and vitamin P are needed, and they are found in any well-balanced diet.

ROUGHAGE

Roughage is the term applied to fibres which are indigestible. They simply pass through the body and in so doing help to eliminate waste products. Constipation arises from lack of roughage in the diet, and if persistent this can lead to colorectal cancer, appendicitis and diverticular disease. These diseases are little known amongst native African tribes whose diet contains coarse grain and other foods rich in fibre. One of the best forms of fibre for the human is cellulose. It is found in both leafy and root vegetables, in fruit, in cereals, and in bran and spinach, which are known to be rich sources. Since cooking softens the fibres and makes them less effective in stimulating elimination, it is best that at least some of the items containing cellulose be eaten raw each day. Perhaps this is the source of the 'apple a day' fable.

OTHER ELEMENTS

The other elements we require to keep our bodies fit are water and air. Our body is composed of between 55 per cent and 70 per cent water, and this fluid must be constantly replenished. We can live for some weeks without food if we have sufficient reserves of fat to draw upon, but we cannot live for more than a few days without water, and not for more than a few seconds without air.

Water is needed for all the cell functions and chemical processes of the body: it dilutes and moistens our food, thereby assisting digestion; it regulates our body temperature through sweating; it helps remove waste products through excretion; it transports those vitamins that are water soluble around our bodies.

We get our water partly in its pure form from the tap or the well, and partly as a constituent of all the other foods we eat. Juicy fruits have a very high water content; even beef has 68 per cent. Foods such as bread and cheese have about 40 per cent. The body requires an intake of at least 4pt ($2\frac{1}{4}$l) a day.

Air is all around us. We breathe not only through our noses but also through our pores. It is vital to afford our bodies as much access to air as possible. Our climate and social customs make nudity impossible, but clothes should be loose fitting and allow our bodies to breathe, and the whole body should be exposed to the air at least for some time during the day whenever possible.

2
The Physical Face of Fitness

It would be out of place in this book to attempt to deal comprehensively with the structure and functioning of our bodies. Such information would fill several books on anatomy and physiology, and can readily be found in such books by those who are interested. In order to guide us in keeping fit, however, it will help to be able to identify our muscles, to know what are normal standards of physical development and performance, and to understand how to correct any deficiencies we may have.

Let us look first at our height and weight measurements. The height we grow to depends on many factors, such as the heights of our parents, housing conditions, access to fresh air and sunshine, the amount of exercise taken, food, and illnesses we or our parents may have had. Today children are regularly weighed at clinics and in school, and mothers will soon learn from the nurse or family doctor if their child is not making the expected progress. For their further information the following guide is given.

Children's Weights

Height	*Boy*	*Girl*
3ft 9in	3st 3lb	3st
3ft 10in	3st 5lb	3st 4lb
3ft 11in	3st 7lb	3st 6lb
4ft	3st 11lb	3st 9lb
4ft 1in	4st	3st 13lb
4ft 2in	4st 1lb	4st
4ft 3in	4st 3lb	4st 1lb
4ft 4in	4st 4lb	4st 3lb
4ft 5in	4st 7lb	4st 5lb
4ft 6in	4st 11lb	4st 9lb
4ft 7in	5st	4st 11lb
4ft 8in	5st 5lb	5st 3lb
4ft 9in	5st 8lb	5st 7lb
4ft 10in	5st 12lb	5st 10lb
4ft 11in	6st 2lb	5st 12lb
5ft	6st 9lb	6st 2lb

These tables must not be taken as rigid levels to be achieved by every child. Much depends on the bone structure of the child, and in judging if he or she is fit, appearance, general health and happiness must be considered as well as weight.

Growth stops at the age of 20 for a girl and 24 for a boy, though weight tends to go on increasing at the rate of ½lb a year up to the age of 50, and if this increase leads to overweight, it must be corrected by diet or exercise or a combination of both.

Adults need not concern themselves unduly with what their height is. Once we have finished growing there is little we can do to increase our height, and if our lack of inches worries us, we must make the most of what we have by good posture. What adults must look at, however, is their weight in relation to their height.

The time to weigh yourself is first thing in the morning, having emptied the bladder. You should get on the scales without clothes on, and at the same time every day, so that gains or losses will be true and not affected by what you have just eaten. The following tables give a general indication of what our weight should be relative to our height when we have reached maturity, ie at 20 for a woman and 24 for the man. The yearly increase mentioned above will add slightly to this as we grow older, but the fitter we are the less will be added.

We must also remember that in addition to height we have to consider bodily type to find out what our weight should be. There are three broad classes of build: the ectomorph, who is the thin, small-boned person; the mesomorph, who is the person of medium build and bone structure; and the endomorph, who is the big-boned, solidly built person. To simplify the tables, I have called them 'small', 'medium' and 'large'.

Weight Table for Men

Height	*Small build*	*Medium build*	*Large build*
5ft 1in	8st	8st 8lb	9st 6lb
5ft 2in	8st 3lb	8st 12lb	9st 9lb
5ft 3in	8st 6lb	9st 1lb	9st 13lb
5ft 4in	8st 9lb	9st 4lb	10st 3lb
5ft 5in	8st 12lb	9st 8lb	10st 7lb
5ft 6in	9st 2lb	9st 12lb	10st 11lb
5ft 7in	9st 6lb	10st 2lb	11st 2lb
5ft 8in	9st 10lb	10st 5lb	11st 6lb
5ft 9in	10st	10st 9lb	11st 11lb
5ft 10in	10st 4lb	11st	12st 2lb
5ft 11in	10st 8lb	11st 4lb	12st 6lb
6ft	10st 12lb	11st 10lb	12st 10lb
6ft 1in	11st 2lb	12st	13st 2lb
6ft 2in	11st 6lb	12st 4lb	13st 8lb
6ft 3in	11st 10lb	12st 8lb	13st 12lb

Weight Table for Women

Height	*Small build*	*Medium build*	*Large build*
4ft 10in	7st	7st 8lb	8st 6lb
4ft 11in	7st 3lb	7st 11lb	8st 9lb
5ft	7st 6lb	8st	8st 12lb
5ft 1in	7st 8lb	8st 4lb	9st 1lb
5ft 2in	7st 11lb	8st 8lb	9st 5lb
5ft 3in	8st	8st 12lb	9st 10lb
5ft 4in	8st 4lb	9st 2lb	9st 13lb
5ft 5in	8st 8lb	9st 4lb	10st 2lb
5ft 6in	8st 12lb	9st 9lb	10st 6lb
5ft 7in	9st 2lb	10st	10st 10lb
5ft 8in	9st 6lb	10st 4lb	11st
5ft 9in	9st 11lb	10st 8lb	11st 4lb
5ft 10in	10st 2lb	10st 11lb	11st 8lb
5ft 11in	10st 4lb	11st	11st 12lb
6ft	10st 8lb	11st 4lb	12st 2lb

It must be emphasised that these or any other tables can only give general indications. A minor deviation in our weight from that shown need cause no alarm. If we can keep round about the weight that is appropriate for our height and build, allowing the slight increase as age advances, we shall know that there is not much wrong with our diet and exercise patterns. All we have to do is to keep up the good work. If we start getting overweight, however, then is the time to start to slim, using the methods indicated in Chapter 5.

We may ask, 'What build can I expect to be?' Wrist measurement in a man or a woman is a good guide to our body type. The small body type will have a 6in wrist; the medium, a 7in wrist; a large, a 7½–8in wrist.

A woman's vital statistics are generally given as bust, waist and hip measurements. Since there are so many variations possible, it is pointless to give figures. Such factors as child bearing can so alter a woman's figure that we would need to know the history of the woman to give meaningful figures. The ideal figure seems to be one in which the bust is one inch less than the hips, and the waist ten inches less than the bust, but fashions change, and such figures indicate aesthetically satisfying proportions rather than fitness or health.

In the case of a man, there are charts of normal development used by weight-trainers for their guidance. At 5ft 8in, a man of small build would have a 38in normal chest, 41in expanded chest, 28in waist, 32in hips and 13½ in flexed biceps. At the same height, a man of medium build would have a 40in normal chest, 42½in expanded chest, 31in waist, 35in hips and 15in flexed biceps. At 5ft 10in, a big man would have a 43in normal chest, 46in expanded chest, 34in waist,

38in hips and 16in flexed biceps. The size of the chest is not as important as the capacity, which is indicated by the difference between normal and expanded measurements.

In addition to weight and measurements, however, we need to consider how agile and supple we are. During the last war, the army brought out a test which was applied to some of their men, indicating the standard of physical performance they found acceptable. It would be useful if we applied a similar, though perhaps less rigorous, test to ourselves.

If you are aged 25, try the following fourteen movements:

1 Run a mile in 7min.

2 Run 100yd in 12sec.

3 Walk 4 miles in 1 hour.

4 Jump forwards (the long jump) to a distance equal to twice your own height.

5 Jump upwards (the high jump) to a distance equal to half your own height.

6 Lift from the ground to the level of your knees a weight equal to your own weight. Be careful to lift correctly by bending your knees and straightening them, so that you avoid strain.

7 Lift to your shoulders a weight equal to 70 per cent of your own bodyweight, and slowly raise it above your head with both hands. This is the movement weight-trainers call 'the press'. If more convenient, try lifting 35 per cent of your bodyweight with one hand above your head, and test each hand in turn.

8 Place both hands on the floor, and keeping the body stiff and straight lower yourself so that the tip of your nose touches the ground and then press yourself back up to arms length again. This is the exercise known as the 'press-up' and is illustrated in Chapter 3 (figs 6a and 6b). Try ten repetitions.

9 Lie on your back and raise your legs slowly to the vertical position, then lower them slowly to the ground again (fig. 31). Try ten repetitions.

10 Lie flat on the floor. Put your feet under something to hold them down. Raise your arms above your head. Now sit up and try to touch your toes (figs. 13a and 13b). Try ten repetitions.

11 Stand upright, hands at sides. Do ten deep knee bends, swinging the arms forwards to shoulder level as you go down and lowering as you come up. Breathe in as you go down and out as you come up (figs. 16a and 16b).

12 Hang by your arms from a beam or a firm branch of a tree and try to pull yourself up to see over

the beam, then lower to arm's length again. (figs 23a and 23b). Try ten repetitions.

13 See if you can touch your toes without bending your knees. Do not strain if you cannot, because the ability is partly dependent on the relative length of your arms and legs and it is a mistake to force yourself beyond what you can naturally do.

14 By bending one arm up your back and taking the other behind your neck, see if you can make the fingers touch behind your back. Again, this is a simple test of suppleness, and do not force yourself if you cannot do it. Weight-trainers and others who develop big shoulder muscles often find difficulty with this.

These fourteen tests are an indication of what a normal 25-year-old should be able to do. They are not the performances of trained athletes to whom they would appear very simple. If you cannot do them, therefore, you are not really as fit as you should be. Older people will need to make some allowances for themselves. Their times for running the mile and the 100 yards will be longer; their time for walking the 4 miles will be longer; they will not be able to jump so high or so far, and their endurance will be less. These tests will have revealed just how far they fall short, however, and they can try to recover lost ground.

In any programme of exercising, the essential thing is to get all-round exercise. Every muscle must get its share of exercise. Too many occupations and even games leave a lot of muscles unused. Runners may have well developed leg muscles and good breathing, but unless their training is all embracing their shoulder and arm muscles may be relatively poorly developed.

In order to facilitate this all-round exercising, it will help to be able to identify the various muscles of the body, so that when we come to the schedules in the later chapters we shall know what we are about.

MUSCLES OF THE BODY

Consult Figs. 1 and 2. Fig. 1 shows the front view of a male body; Fig. 2 a rear view. As far as the main muscle groups to be exercised are concerned, the female structure is similar, though some muscle groups will be more prominently developed in one sex than the other.

Stand stripped in front of a mirror and try to identify on your own body the muscles listed. If they are poorly developed they may not be easy to pick out. The same will be true if you are very stout, as the

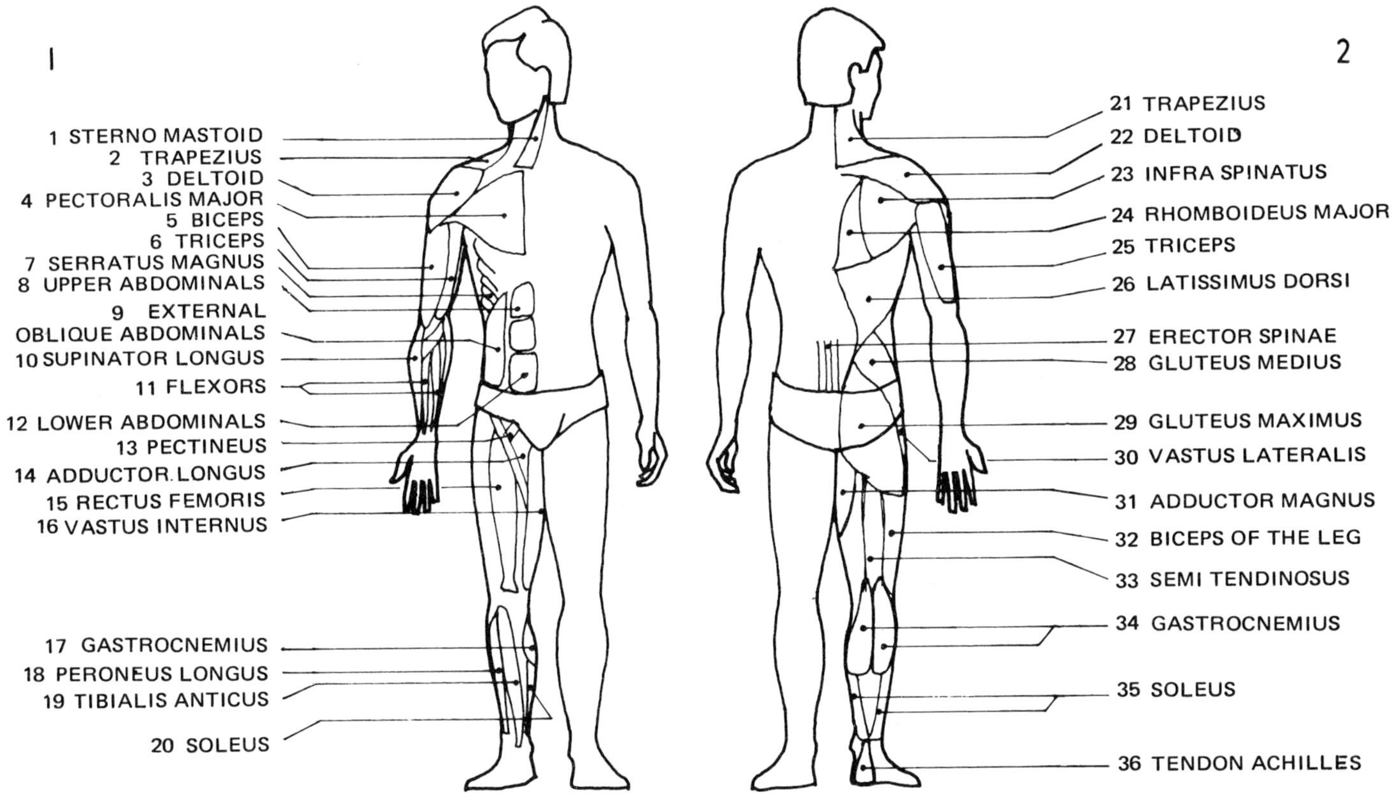
1
2
1 STERNO MASTOID
2 TRAPEZIUS
3 DELTOID
4 PECTORALIS MAJOR
5 BICEPS
6 TRICEPS
7 SERRATUS MAGNUS
8 UPPER ABDOMINALS
9 EXTERNAL OBLIQUE ABDOMINALS
10 SUPINATOR LONGUS
11 FLEXORS
12 LOWER ABDOMINALS
13 PECTINEUS
14 ADDUCTOR LONGUS
15 RECTUS FEMORIS
16 VASTUS INTERNUS
17 GASTROCNEMIUS
18 PERONEUS LONGUS
19 TIBIALIS ANTICUS
20 SOLEUS
21 TRAPEZIUS
22 DELTOID
23 INFRA SPINATUS
24 RHOMBOIDEUS MAJOR
25 TRICEPS
26 LATISSIMUS DORSI
27 ERECTOR SPINAE
28 GLUTEUS MEDIUS
29 GLUTEUS MAXIMUS
30 VASTUS LATERALIS
31 ADDUCTOR MAGNUS
32 BICEPS OF THE LEG
33 SEMI TENDINOSUS
34 GASTROCNEMIUS
35 SOLEUS
36 TENDON ACHILLES

layers of fat will hide them. Try at least to see where they lie, and to understand what each muscle is used for, as this knowledge will be invaluable to you when you come to the exercises themselves.

THE TRAPEZIUS

This muscle covers the shoulder and the upper part of the back of the neck. It is number 2 on Fig. 1 and number 21 on Fig. 2. It helps in all movements of the shoulder joint, such as lifting something up in front of you, and it also enables you to square your shoulders and to take your head back.

THE STERNO-MASTOIDS

These are the muscles at the sides of your neck (*see* number 1 in Fig. 1). They enable you to turn your head from side to side or to lift up and down.

THE DELTOIDS

These are the bands of muscles that cover the shoulder joint (number 3 in Fig. 1 and number 22 in Fig. 2). They enable you to raise your arms sideways or to raise them straight up in front of you.

THE PECTORALIS MAJOR

These are the big triangular muscles on the front of your chest (number 4 in Fig. 1). They can most readily be seen on the male by placing the hands on the hips and dropping the shoulders slightly forward. They enable you to move your arms forwards and also to pull them into your body.

THE BICEPS

These are the large muscles at the front of the top of the arms (number 5 in Fig. 1). They enable you to bend your arm at the elbow joint.

THE TRICEPS

These are the muscles at the back of the upper arm (number 6 in Fig. 1 and number 25 in Fig. 2). They enable you to straighten your arm.

SERRATUS MAGNUS

These are the little ridges of muscle that can be seen on the sides of your body under your armpits (number 7 in Fig. 1). They enable you to lift your arm sideways.

THE SUPINATOR LONGUS

This is the muscle at the side and back of your forearm (number 10 in Fig. 1). It enables you to turn your wrist from side to side.

FLEXORS

These are the muscles at the front of your forearm (number 11 in Fig. 1). They enable you to bend your wrist inwards.

THE EXTERNAL OBLIQUE ABDOMINALS

These muscles extend from the lower ribs down the sides of your body (number 9 in Fig. 1). They enable you to turn your body from side to side, to bend sideways and to straighten up again.

THE UPPER AND LOWER ABDOMINALS

These muscles at the front of your body extend from the lower ribs to the pubic bone (numbers 8 and 12 in Fig. 1). They enable you to bend forwards, to raise your legs straight out in front of you and to sit up when you are lying flat.

THE PECTINEUS AND THE ADDUCTOR LONGUS

These muscles are on the inside of the upper thigh (numbers 13 and 14 in Fig. 1). They move the thigh inwards.

THE RECTUS FEMORIS

This is the long muscle running down the front of the thigh (number 15 in Fig. 1). It is used in movements from the hip joint, such as raising the leg forwards, or straightening the leg out in front of you when the knee is raised.

THE VASTUS INTERNUS

This is the muscle at the side and back of your upper leg (number 16 in Fig. 1). It enables you to turn your leg.

THE PERONEUS LONGUS

This is the muscle at the side of your lower leg (number 18 in Fig. 1). Together with other muscles in this area of the body, it enables you to move the foot and rotate the leg.

THE TIBIALIS ANTICUS

This is the big muscle at the front of your calf (number 19 in Fig. 1). It helps you bend the foot upwards.

THE GASTROCNEMIUS AND THE SOLEUS

These muscles are at the side and back of your calf (number 17 and 20 in Fig. 1 and numbers 34 and 35 in Fig. 2). The gastrocnemius flexes the foot, so that you can bend it backwards; the main function of the soleus is to enable you to maintain an upright posture.

THE INFRA SPINATUS AND THE RHOMBOIDEUS MAJOR

These muscles are at the back of your shoulder (numbers 23 and 24 in Fig. 2). They enable you to take your shoulders back, and they assist with such actions as pulling.

THE LATISSIMUS DORSI

This is the large muscle at the back of your body (number 26 in Fig. 2). It enables you to rotate the body and to raise the arms at the shoulder joint.

THE ERECTOR SPINAE

This is the muscle group in the small of your back (number 27 in Fig. 2). They enable you to straighten the back after bending forwards.

THE GLUTEUS MEDIUS AND THE GLUTEUS MAXIMUS

These are the fleshy muscles of the buttocks (numbers 28 and 29 in Fig. 2). They enable you to rotate and move the legs.

THE VASTUS LATERALIS

This is the muscle at the side and back of your upper leg (number 30 in Fig. 2). It enables you to raise the leg sideways from the hip joint and assists in bending the knee.

THE ADDUCTOR MAGNUS

This is the muscle at the back of the inside of the upper leg (number 31 in Fig. 2). It enables you to turn the leg, as in pointing the foot outwards.

THE BICEPS OF THE LEG AND THE SEMI-TENDINOSUS

These two muscles are at the back of the upper leg (numbers 32 and 33 in Fig. 2). They fulfil a similar function in the leg as the biceps do in the arm, enabling you to bend your knee and so bring your leg backwards.

THE ACHILLES TENDON

This is a tendon which is a tough fibrous substance joining a muscle to a bone not a muscle and is located at the base of the back of the leg. Its function is to insert the gastrocnemius muscle into the calcaneum (number 36 in Fig. 2).

All the muscles listed here are known as 'voluntary muscles' because they can be moved at will. We can develop them by exercise, and later in the book we shall learn how. We also have a vast number of involuntary muscles, the heart being a common and well-known example. These involuntary muscles do not respond to conscious effort, and therefore we cannot exert any influence on their development. But we can keep them fit by attention to our general state of health.

3
Daily Exercises

Most people, at some time or another, think that they ought to take more exercise. They are quite right. One of the reasons why the thought is often not put into action is that they simply do not know what exercises to do. The more resolute may end up by walking to work instead of taking the car, and this is helpful in its way but not good enough to keep them really fit, since it exercises only some of their muscles, not all.

To keep the body truly fit we must have all-round exercise, so that each muscle is worked on in turn and kept in good condition. In this chapter we shall consider how to exercise, when, and what to do.

HOW SHOULD WE EXERCISE?

We should exercise in a warm room in winter, but with the window open to allow plenty of fresh air. In summer exercise can beneficially be done in the open air. The ideal is to wear as little as possible, and any clothes we do wear should be loose and not restrict our movements. Bra and slacks are suitable for a woman, and trunks for a man, or even complete nudity if we have privacy. There are three reasons for not wearing much:

1 The body breathes through the pores of the skin as well as the nose, and needs unrestricted access to oxygen when we exercise.

2 Belts or other tight garments may restrict our movements in the wrong way, so leading to our being unable to make a full, free movement, with possible risk of strain.

3 We need to watch what we are doing to get the maximum benefit from our exercise, and for this reason we should exercise in front of a large mirror.

We have learnt in Chapter 2 how to identify our muscles, in this chapter we shall be told which muscles are being used in each exercise. Concentrate on them by watching their action in the mirror. This not only helps to make sure you are doing the exercise correctly, it actually benefits the muscle. Weight-trainers have proved that it really assists development. The reason why a manual worker is not always as well developed as a weight-trainer is this lack of concentration. The worker is thinking about the job in hand; the weight-trainer about the muscles used.

WHEN SHOULD WE EXERCISE?

You should exercise at the same time every day. Evening will probably be the most convenient time for many people, but you must allow an hour and a half to elapse after your evening meal. It may be more convenient to do your exercises when you undress for bed; they could then be followed by a bath or shower before you lie down. For the purpose of keeping fit the schedule of exercises in this chapter could be followed daily. If, however, you are aiming to develop certain muscles of your body so as to correct under-development you do not need daily exercise. You need more rigorous schedules to be followed every other day, and should consult Chapter 6. For general health and fitness, however, follow the routine in this chapter daily.

WHAT EXERCISES SHOULD WE DO?

The following routine uses no apparatus except what would be found in a normal house, yet it covers all the muscle groups in turn and will provide an all-round work-out, toning up the muscles and developing suppleness and grace of movement. We begin and end with very important breathing exercises. Start your training with these sixteen movements.

EXERCISE 1 DEEP BREATHING

Stand upright and relaxed, feet normal distance apart, head up and chest forward. Cross the arms in front of you with palms facing in towards your body (Fig. 3a). Breathe out so that you empty your lungs as much as possible. Now, slowly uncross your arms and take them up and backwards above your shoulders, filling your lungs with a deep breath as you do so (Fig. 3b).

When you have drawn in as much oxygen as you can, slowly bring the arms back to the first position, breathing out as you do so. Concentrate on emptying the lungs and they will fill themselves when you breathe in (Fig. 3c).

Do ten repetitions.

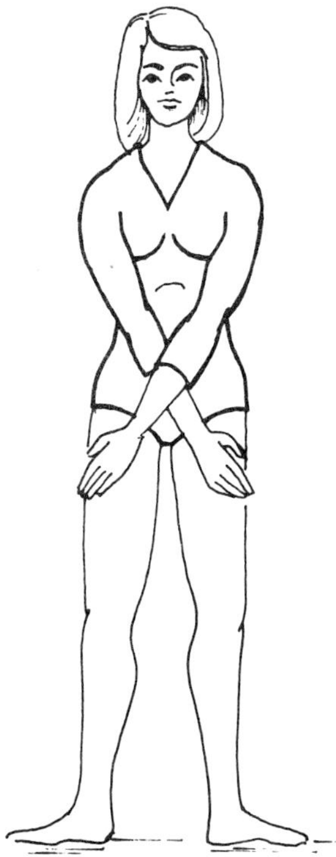

3a

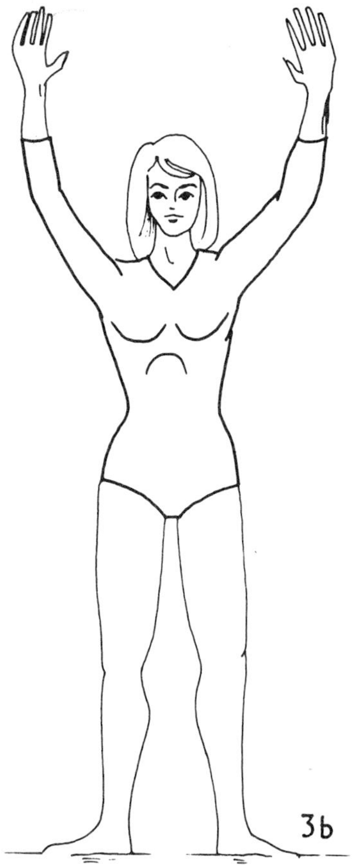

3b

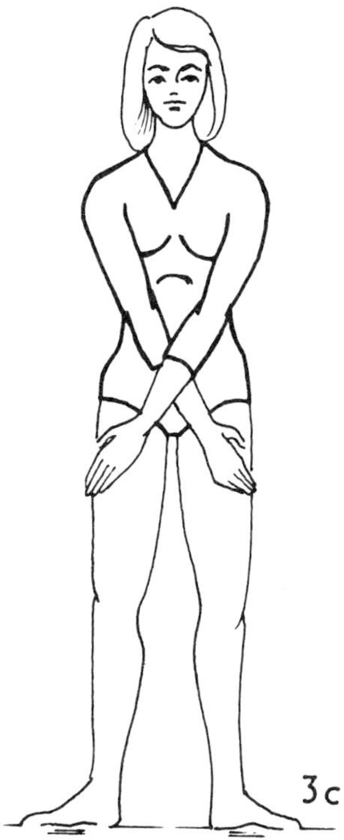

3c

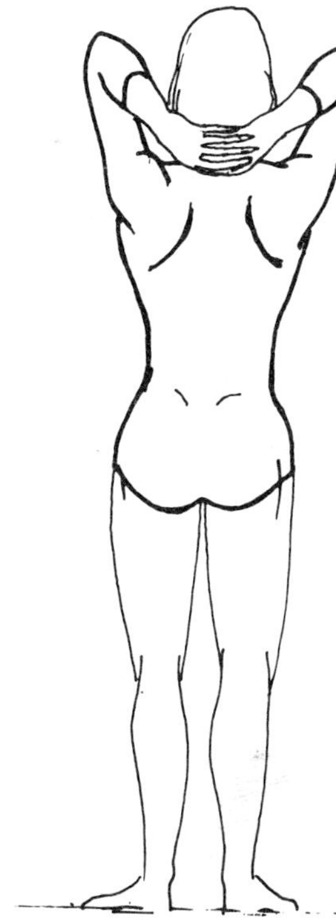

4

EXERCISE 2 FOR THE NECK MUSCLES

Clasp the hands behind the back of the head and bring the elbows forward (Fig. 4). Now pull the head forward with your hands with a slow, gentle pressure and at the same time resist the pull by pushing back with your head. Your head does not move in fact; it is held stationary by the opposing forces. The effort is good for the trapezius muscles in particular.

Do ten repetitions.

EXERCISE 3 FOR THE STERNO-MASTOIDS

Stand upright and relaxed. Turn the head to look over the left shoulder as far as possible without straining (Fig. 5a). Now turn the head the other way to look as far as possible over your right shoulder, again without straining (Fig. 5b).

Do ten repetitions each side.

EXERCISE 4 FOR THE ARMS, SHOULDERS, BACK AND CHEST

This exercise is such an all-round one that it is almost a complete training schedule on its own. In addition to the obvious benefits to the muscles mentioned, it is

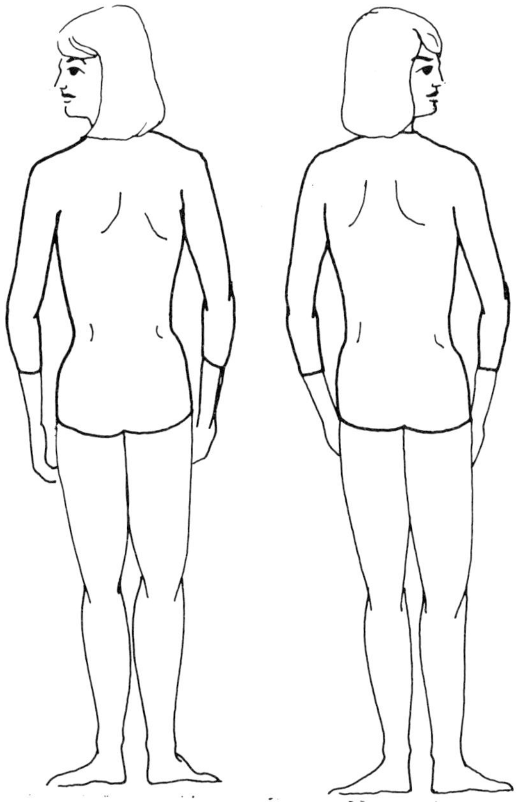

5a 5b

6a

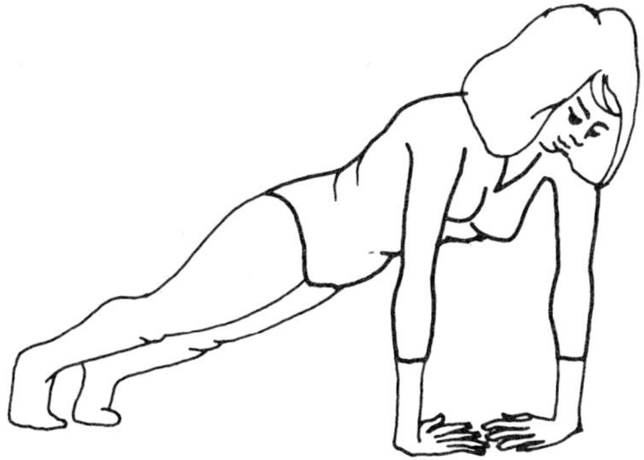

6b

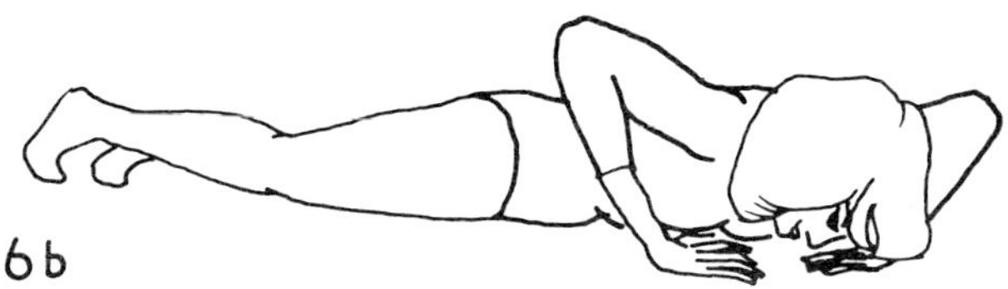

beneficial to the abdominal muscles through the control of the body which must be exercised.

Place the hands on the floor, shoulder width apart, fingers pointing inwards. Stretch out the body so that the toes are on the floor with the body held in a straight line (Fig. 6a). Now lower the body so that the nose touches the floor, holding the body rigid all the time. Breathe in as you go down. This brings you to position 6b. Press yourself back up to the position in Fig. 6a by straightening your arms. Breathe out as you do so. Lower again, breathing in.

Do ten repetitions. If you cannot manage ten repetitions at first, do as many as you can and try to add one a week until your number reaches 10. If, in the beginning, you find that you simply cannot do the exercise at all, try lowering yourself just a little way, and then a little farther the next time, until you are able to complete the movement.

EXERCISE 5 FOR THE DELTOIDS

Hold the back of a chair which is facing away from you (Fig. 7a). Note that you grasp the bar at the back of the chair from above, with your palms towards yourself. Now raise the chair to shoulder level, breathing out as you do so (the position to which you raise the chair is shown in Fig. 7b). Then lower the chair, breathing in as you do so. Do ten repetitions.

EXERCISE 6 FOR THE BICEPS

For this you will need a weight of some kind. The old type of flat iron with a handle would be suitable, and a dumb-bell would be ideal. Equally a book, a brick or a heavy plastic bag filled with earth or sand would do.

Stand upright; take the weight in your right hand, palm facing the front, arm hanging loosely at your side (Fig. 8a). Now raise the weight to your shoulder level by slowly bending your arm (Fig. 8b). Breathe out as you do so.

Lower the weight to your side again, breathing in as you do so. The left arm should be hanging by your left side as you do the exercise with your right arm, palm flat against your left side.

Do ten repetitions slowly with the right arm, then change over and do ten with the left.

I would emphasise that the movement must be done slowly. It is fairly easy if done quickly, but it is the slow, controlled movement that exercises the muscle best and which will make you feel the effect afterwards in the form of a mild ache.

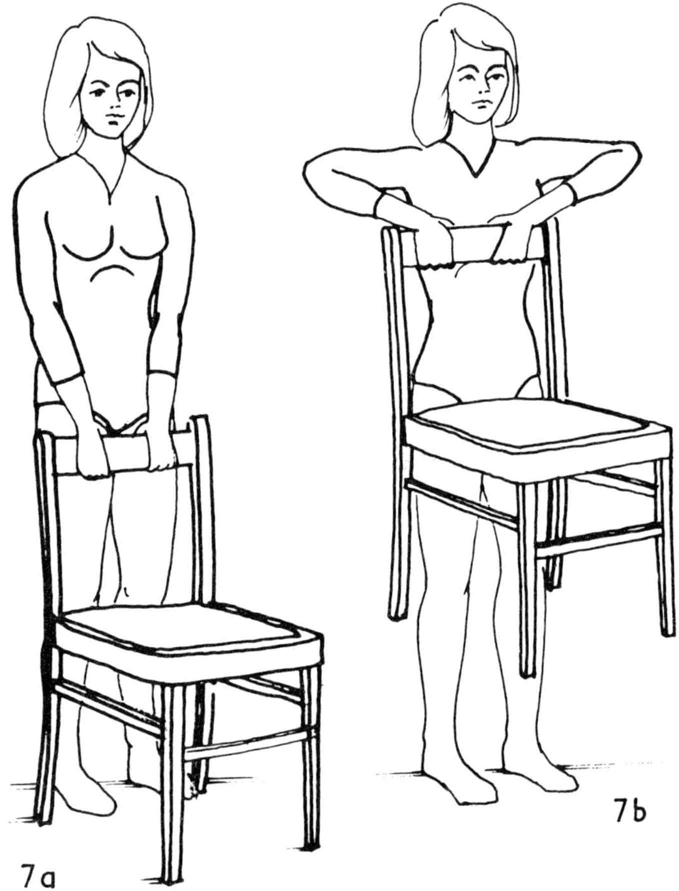

7a 7b

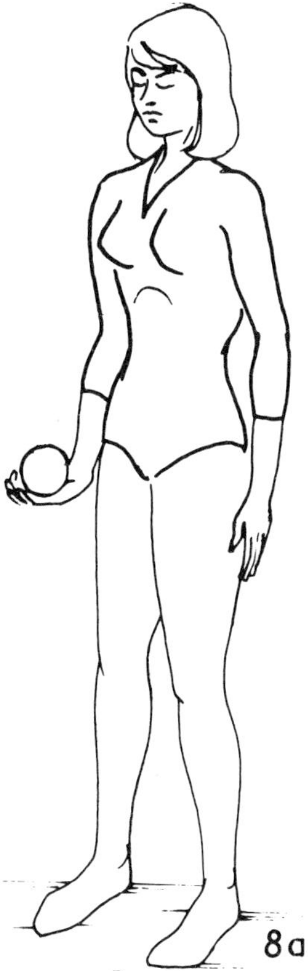

8a

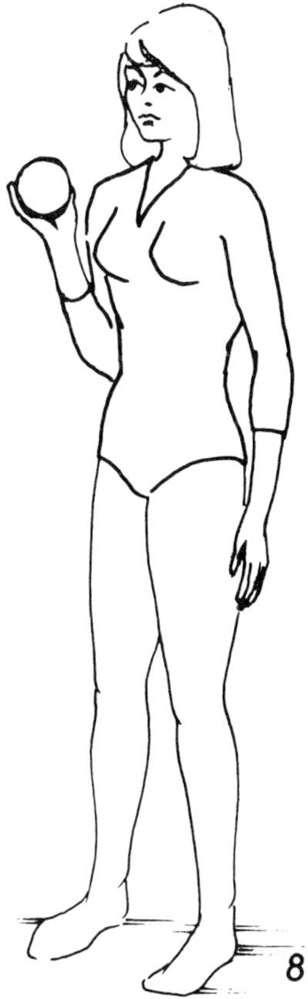

8b

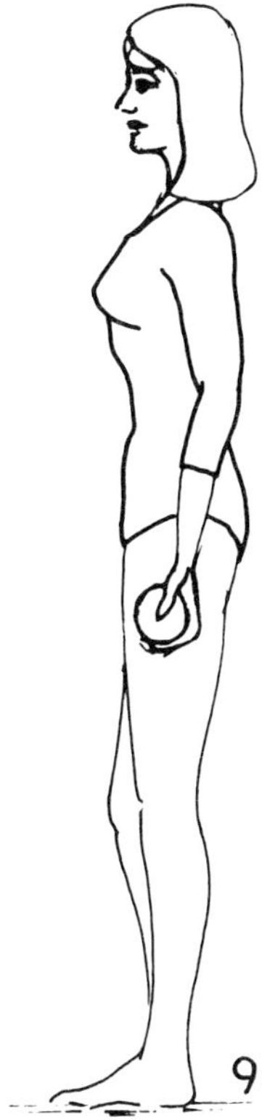

9a

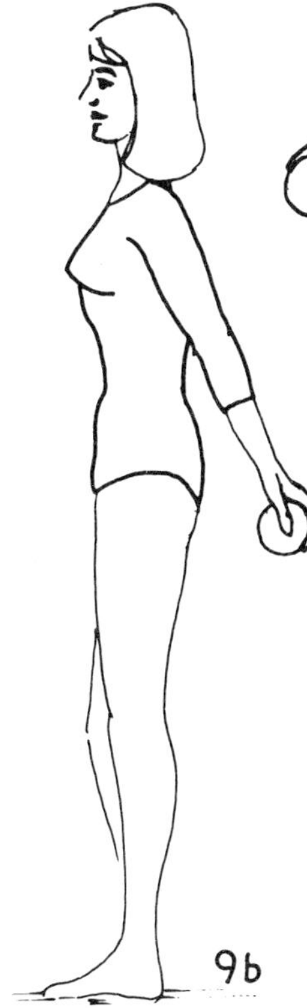

9b

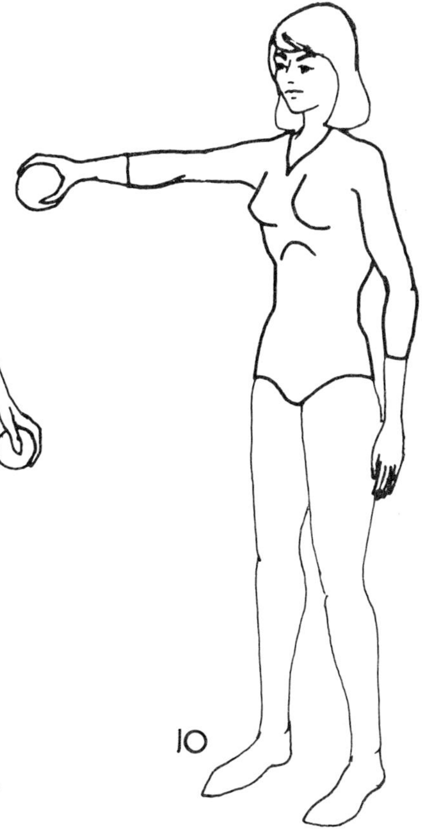

10

EXERCISE 7 FOR THE TRICEPS

This again is best done with a weight such as you used in the last movement. Remember that the biceps are the muscles in the front of your upper arm used when you bend the elbow, and the triceps are the muscles at the back used when you straighten the arm.

Let your left hand hang loosely by your side, holding your weight with palm to the front as before (Fig. 9a). Now slowly raise the arm backwards as far as it will go, keeping the body upright, with the palm of the hand to the front and the back of the hand to the rear. Keep your right hand by your side as you are doing the exercise with your left. Breathe out as you raise the arm, in as you lower it (Fig. 9b).

Do ten repetitions with the left arm and ten with the right.

EXERCISE 8 FOR THE WRIST

Take a rubber ball, such as a tennis ball, and hold it out at arm's length in front of you with your right hand, palm downwards (Fig. 10). Alternatively squeeze the ball with the hand and then relax.

Do ten movements with the right hand, and then ten with the left.

EXERCISE 9 FOR THE SIDE ABDOMINALS

Stand upright, feet apart, arms hanging loosely at your sides (Fig. 11a). Bend over to your right, letting your right palm slide down the side of your right leg and bringing your left fist up under your left armpit (Fig. 11b). Straighten up and move smoothly over to your left, with your left palm sliding down the side of your left leg and your right fist coming up under your right armpit (Fig. 11c).

Alternate in a smooth, flowing movement. Try to reach a little farther down the leg each time, but do not strain. Do twenty bends to each side.

EXERCISE 10 FOR THE ABDOMINALS

Stand upright, arms held straight out in line with the shoulders (Fig. 12a). Turn as far as possible to your right, keeping your arms out straight (Fig. 12b). Turn back to the front and straight round as far as possible to the left in a smooth, swinging action (Fig. 12c).

Do twenty turns to each side, going as far round as possible. Both in this exercise and in the one before you will feel the pull in the muscles at the sides of your body.

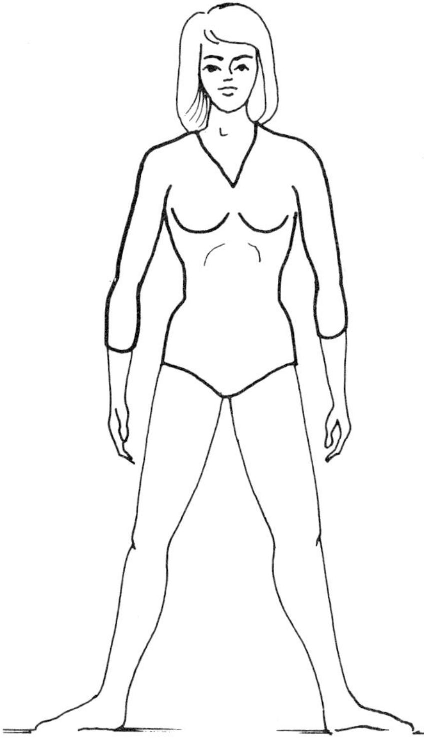

11a

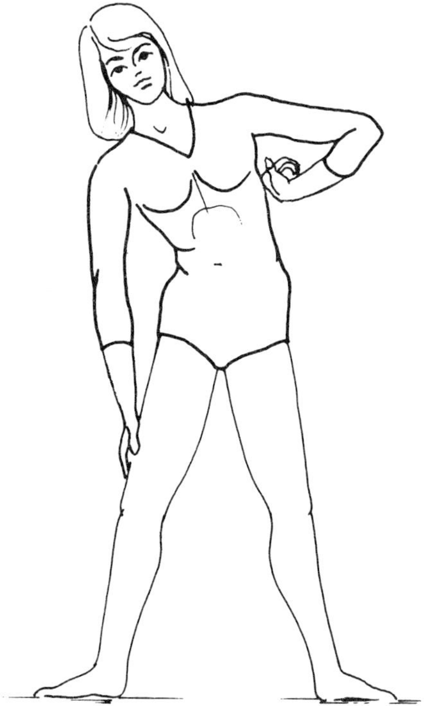

11b

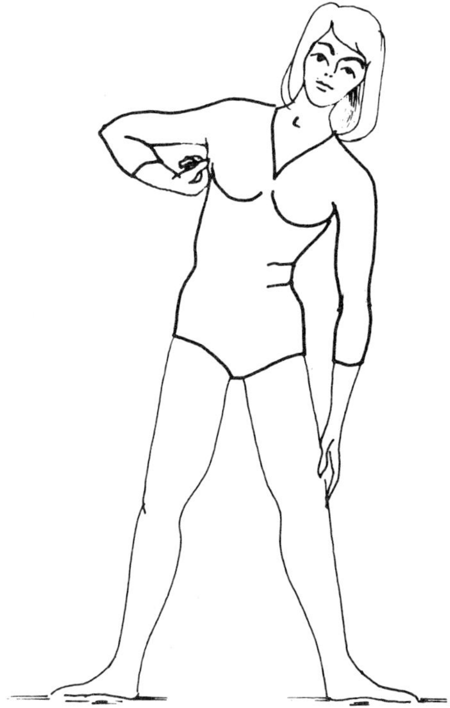

11c

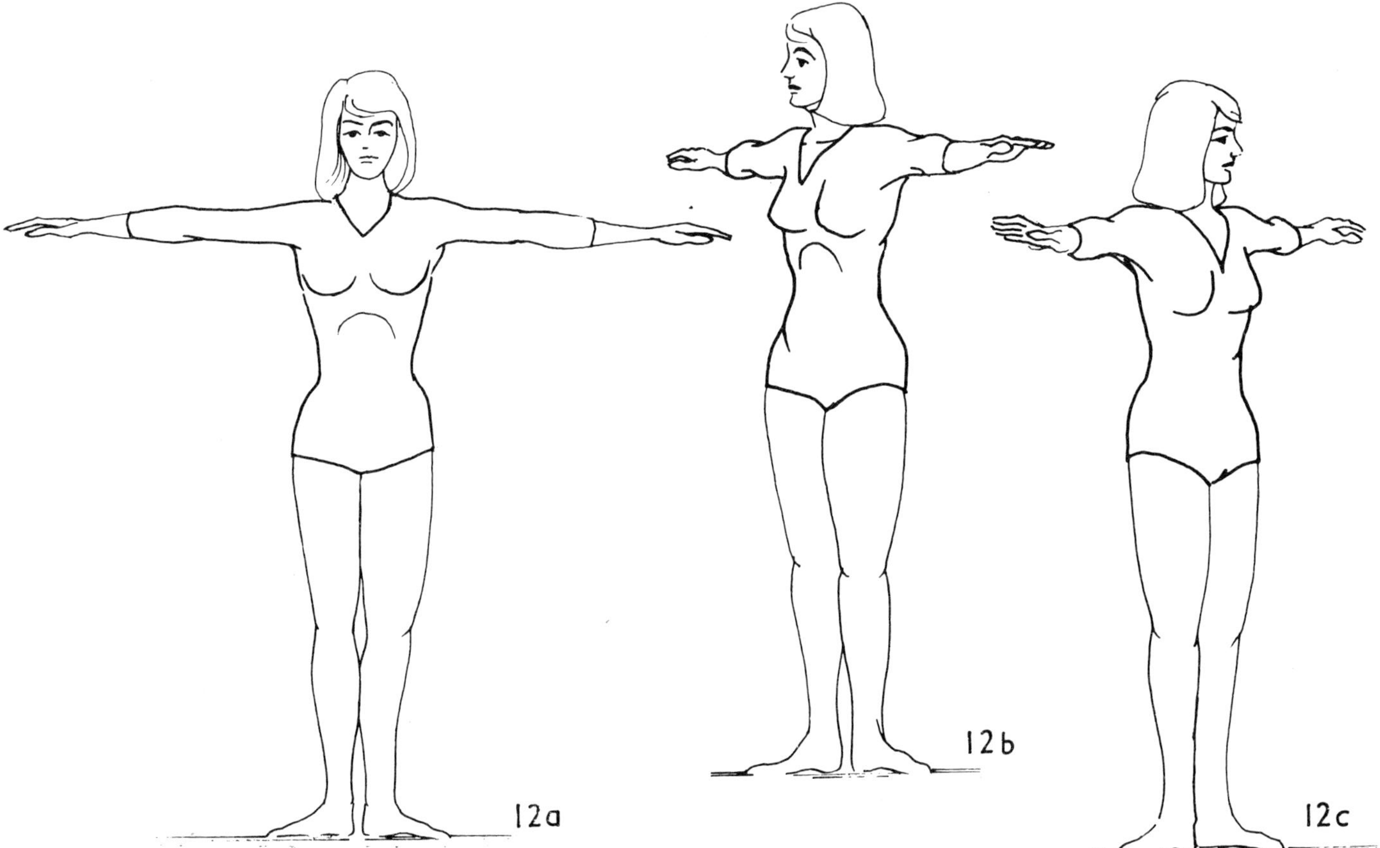

12a 12b 12c

EXERCISE 11 FOR THE UPPER ABDOMINALS

Lie flat on the floor, arms above your head (Fig. 13a). It is best for this exercise if you can tuck your feet under something, such as a heavy chair, or get someone to hold them down, or failing either of these things, place a heavy cushion on them. What you have to do is to sit up and touch your toes (Fig. 13b).

Breathe out as you sit up and in as you lower back to the first position. You must try to do the exercise slowly, controlling your body, particularly when you lower. You will not find this easy. Initially you may need a little swing of the arms to give you the impetus to come up, but try to progress to doing it without this aid, so that the abdominal muscles do the work. Try to lower yourself back slowly and not flop back even from the beginning.

Do ten repetitions.

EXERCISE 12 FOR THE LOWER ABDOMINALS

Again lie flat on your back, but this time with arms at your sides and palms on the ground (Fig. 14a). Raise both heels slightly off the ground, about one inch. Now slowly raise the left leg as high as it will go, keeping the right heel about an inch off the ground as you do so (Fig. 14b). Then lower the left leg and raise the right at the same time. Do not put the left heel back on the ground, but stop when it is one inch off the ground (Fig. 14c).

Do ten repetitions with each leg before allowing the heels to touch the floor again.

In the beginning you may not be able to do this. In that case, do the same exercise but without taking the heels off the floor. This will not benefit your abdominal muscles as much, of course, and as soon as you can progress to doing the exercise properly you must do so.

EXERCISE 13 FOR THE BACK

Stand with the feet wide apart, arms above the head (Fig. 15a). Now bend forwards and try to touch the ground in front of you and between the legs (Fig. 15b). Breathe out as you go down and in as you come up. Do not bend the knees. If you cannot touch the ground in the beginning, go as far as you can but do not strain or force yourself, as the ability depends as much on the length of the arm relative to the leg as on suppleness, and the old idea they had in schools of forcing children to touch their toes has now been seen to result in

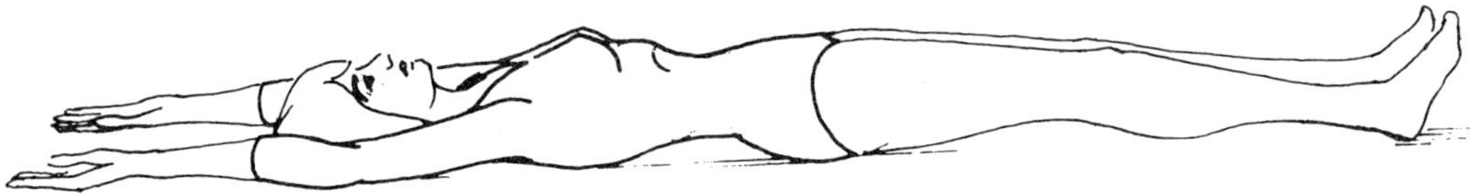

13a

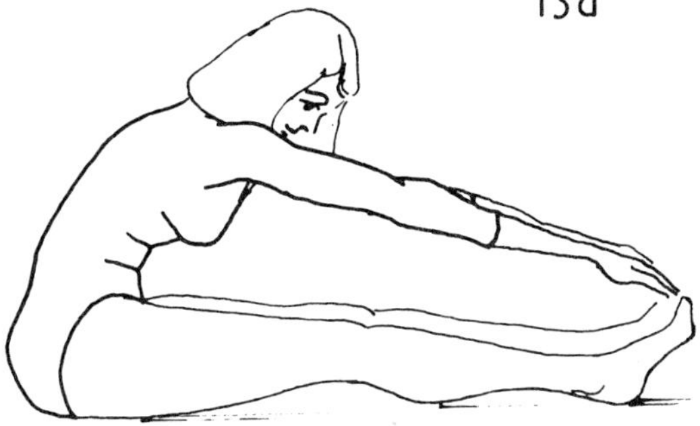

13b

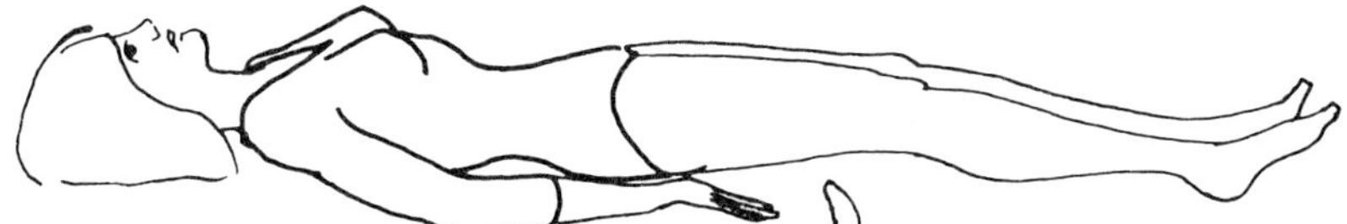

14a

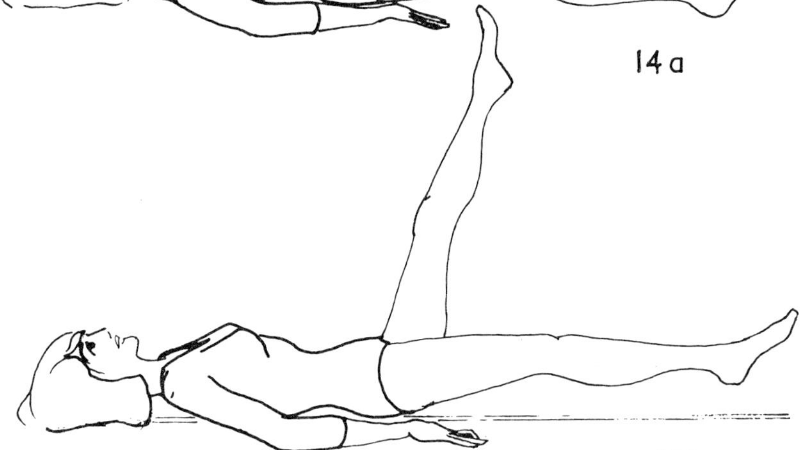

14b

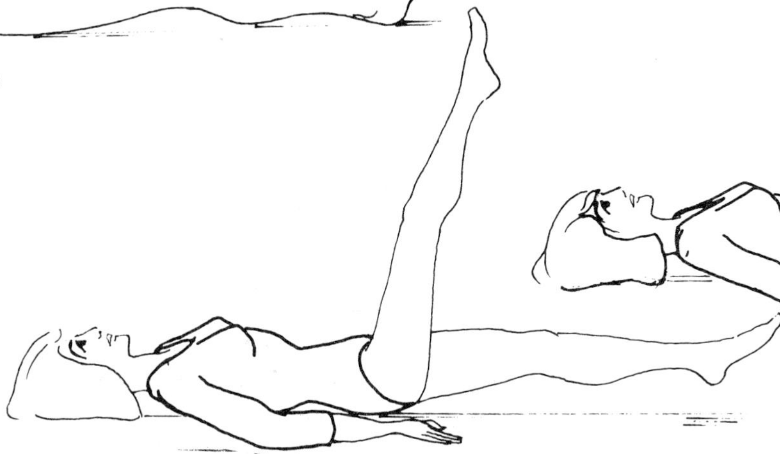

14c

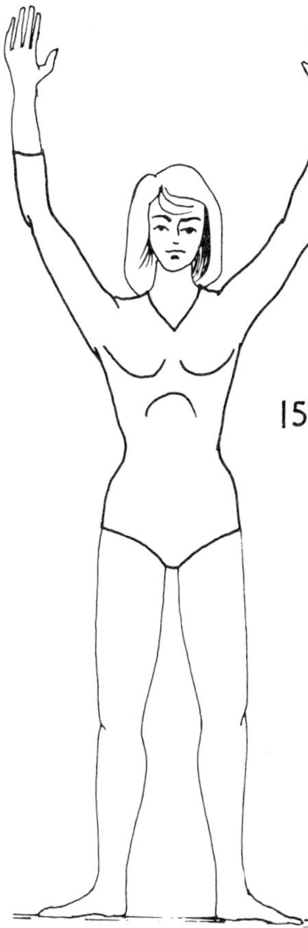

15a

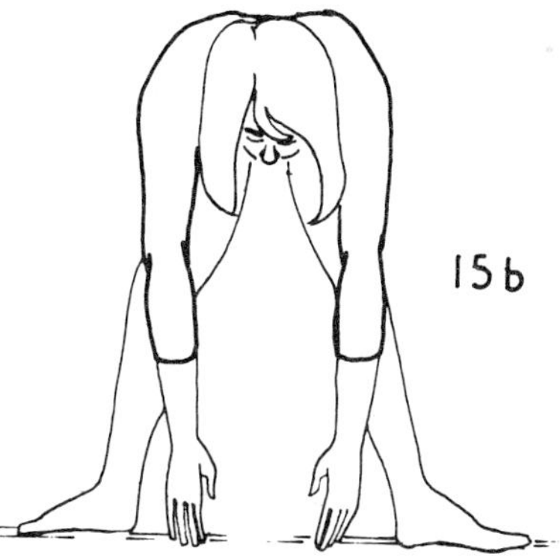

15b

spinal weakness in later life.

Do ten repetitions in a smooth, swinging motion.

EXERCISE 14 FOR THE LEG MUSCLES

Stand upright, heels together, hands at your sides (Fig. 16a). Bend the knees and lower the body, keeping upright, and as you do so swing your arms out in front of you to shoulder level (Fig. 16b). Breathe in as you go down. Come back up by straightening the knees, breathing out as you do so and lowering the arms to the sides.

In this exercise you may raise the heels if you wish, but when you are more experienced try to keep them flat on the ground, as this will be beneficial to the ankle joint, making it more supple.

Do twenty repetitions.

EXERCISE 15 FOR THE ANKLES

Sit cross-legged on the ground. Take your right leg in your right hand just above the ankle. Take the right foot in the left hand (Fig. 17). Now hold the right leg still with the right hand, and gently rotate the foot on the ankle joint with the left hand, first in a clockwise direction and then anti-clockwise. Be careful not to strain. Change over and do the same exercise on the left ankle by holding the left leg in the left hand and the left foot in the right hand.

Do ten repetitions each way.

This exercise may appear very simple, but it is used by karate masters to strengthen the joint and to make it more supple, and is of very real benefit.

EXERCISE 16 DEEP BREATHING

End your training session by repeating number 1. This not only relaxes you but is beneficial in itself in developing the chest and lungs.

This simple routine will have exercised every important muscle group in your body from top to toe and will take up no more than fifteen to twenty minutes of your time each day. Do not be deceived by the fact that these are all well-known exercises and quite simple movements. There is no virtue in trying unusual or original exercises when there are well-tried and proven ones which are just as good.

Concentrate on your exercises and try to understand which muscles are being used. You will probably feel

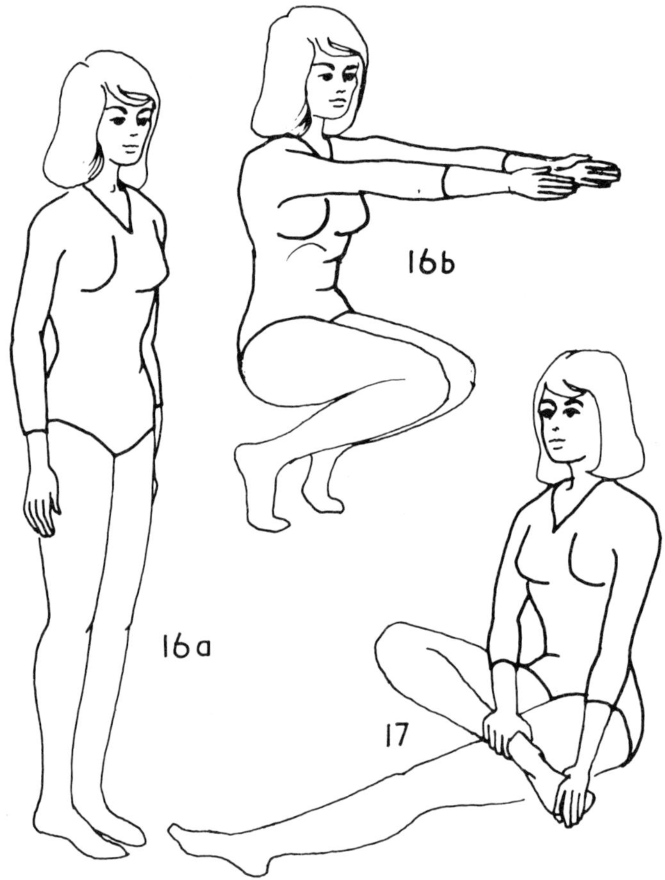

a gentle ache in them the next day. Do not be worried or let this put you off. The aching means that the exercise has done you good.

Although it has just been said that there is no virtue in original or unusual exercises for originality's sake, it is none-the-less a fact that people get tired of doing the same exercises every day. When you feel the need for a change, therefore, you may substitute variations. Variations on all sixteen exercises are given below and numbers indicate which exercise each variation is intended to replace. You must be careful to use them correctly and only use them as substitutes for the correct ones in the original schedule, so that you maintain an all-round programme of exercises.

There is a great temptation to do those exercises that you like and to omit the others. The ones you like are generally those you find easiest, and hence are the ones you least need, since the ease is attributable to the fact that the muscles being used are already fairly well-developed. It is the exercises you do not like because you find them difficult that do you the most good, since they work on your underdeveloped areas to improve them.

Substitute correctly, therefore, and be firm with yourself.

VARIATIONS ON EXERCISE 1

1 Stand upright, arms held straight out in front of you at shoulder level (Fig. 18a). Swing the arms back and press the shoulders back, breathing in deeply as you do so (Fig. 18b). Bring the arms forward to the position in Fig. 18a, breathing out as you do so.

Do ten repetitions.

2 Stand with your back against a wall and your heels about one foot from the wall (Fig. 19). Put your hands flat on your stomach. Breathe in deeply, pressing in and up with your hands. Breathe out as you relax the pressure with your hands. Keep your back flat against the wall.

Do ten repetitions.

VARIATION ON EXERCISE 2

Stand upright and relaxed. Lower the head forwards as far as possible, dropping the chin towards the neck. Now slowly take it up and back as far as possible, so that you are looking up at the ceiling. Do not strain, but perform the movement slowly with concentration.

Do ten repetitions.

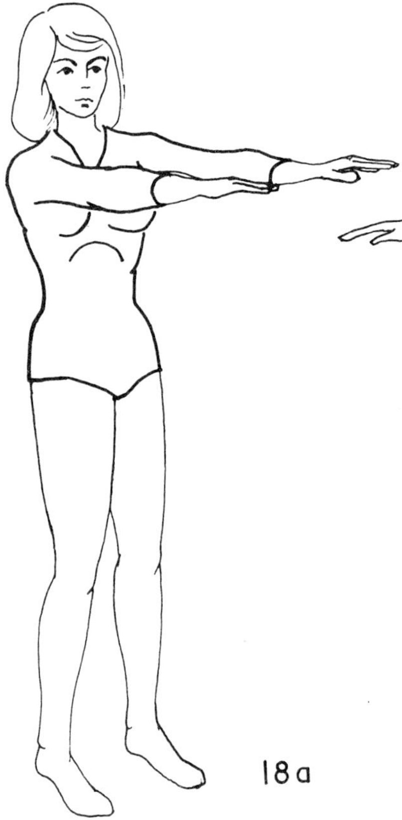

18a

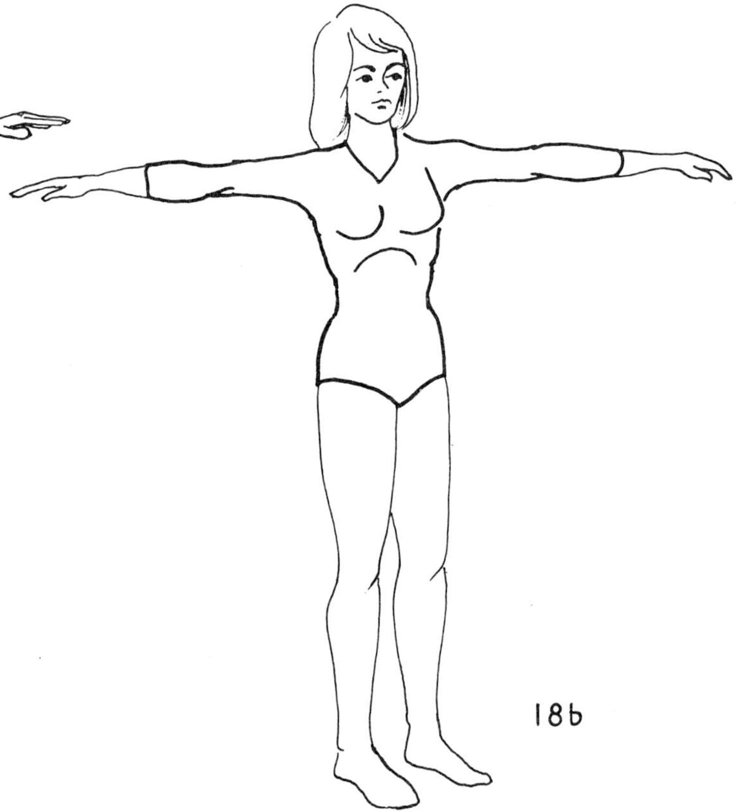

18b

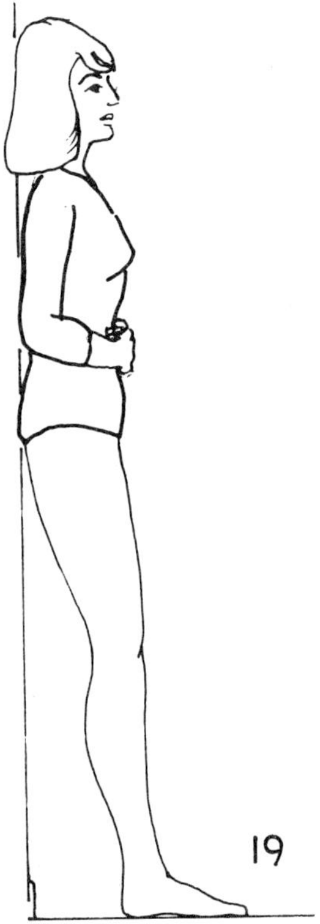

19

20a

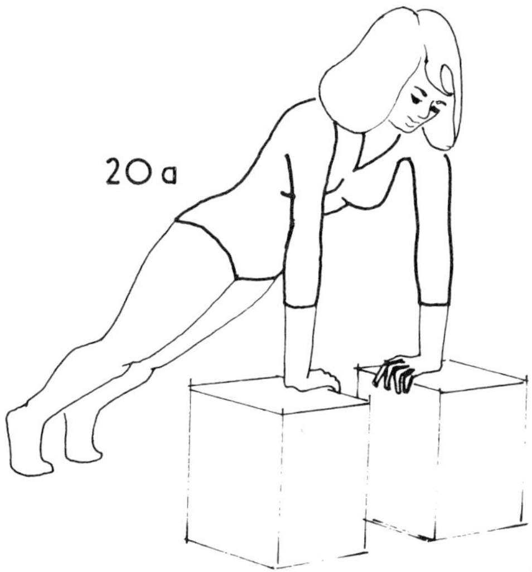

20b

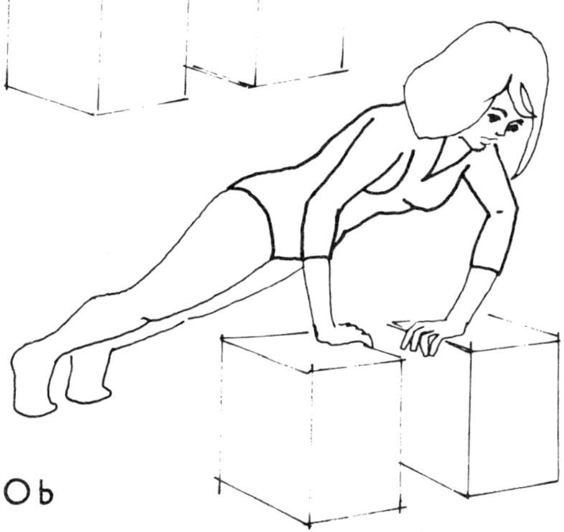

VARIATION ON EXERCISE 3

Bend the head as far to the left as possible, taking the ear down towards the shoulder. Then slowly bring it upright again and over towards the right, taking the right ear down towards the right shoulder. Do not strain but perform the movement slowly with concentration.

Do ten repetitions.

VARIATIONS ON EXERCISE 4

1 Place two stools or chairs side by side, with the backs outwards, the seats facing inwards and about the width of your shoulders apart. Place the palms of your hands on the seats; hold the body rigid with the toes on the ground (Fig. 20a).

From this position lower the body as far as possible, breathing in as you do so (Fig. 20b). Press the body back up to the straight-arm position, breathing out as you do so.

Do ten repetitions.

2 Place two chairs side by side, with the backs facing inwards and the width of your shoulders apart. If need be, put a weight on the seat of each chair to hold it stable. Support yourself by placing one hand on

each chair back and take both feet off the ground, bending the feet up behind you (Fig. 21a). From here lower the body as far as possible, breathing in as you do so (Fig. 21b). Press yourself back up to the straight-arm position, breathing out as you do so.

Do ten repetitions.

VARIATION ON EXERCISE 5

Take a suitable heavy object in both hands, with hands close together in front of you and arms straight and close to your body. A loaded shopping basket will be suitable for this exercise (Fig. 22a). Raise it to shoulder level, bringing the hands up to the chin (Fig. 22b). Breathe out as you raise it and in as you lower again.

Do ten repetitions.

VARIATIONS ON EXERCISE 6

1 If you have a bar or a beam from which you can hang to pull yourself up this is an excellent variation on exercise 6. A branch of a tree in the garden would be suitable, or a beam in the garage.

Assuming you can use something suitable, take a

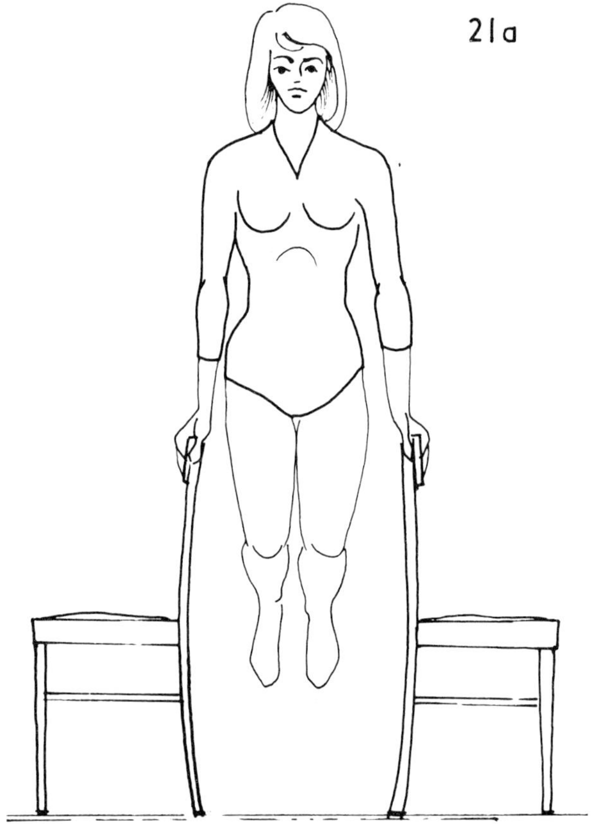

21a

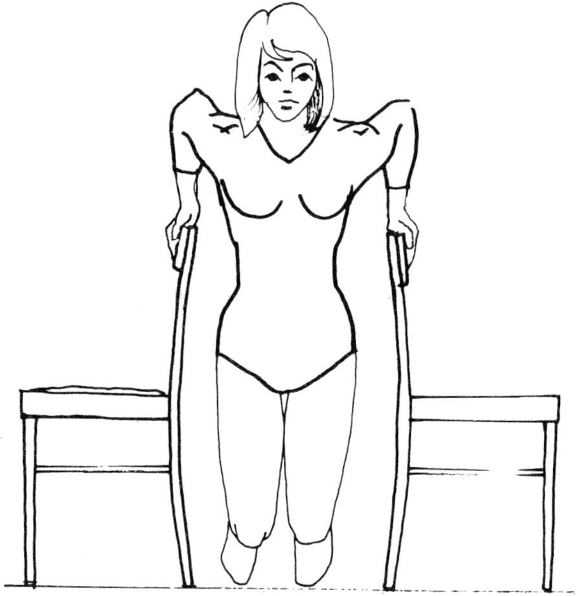

21b

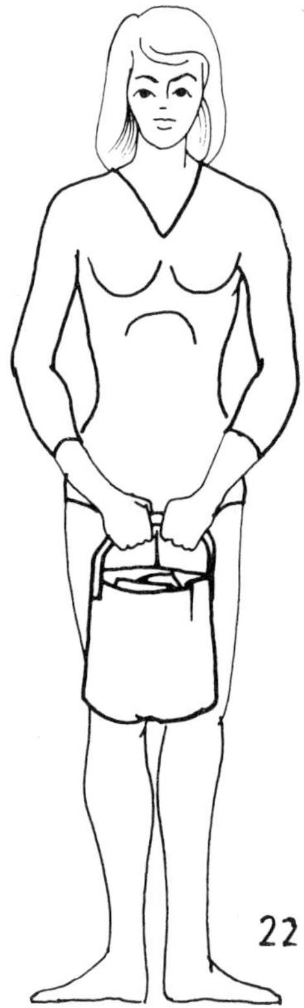

22a

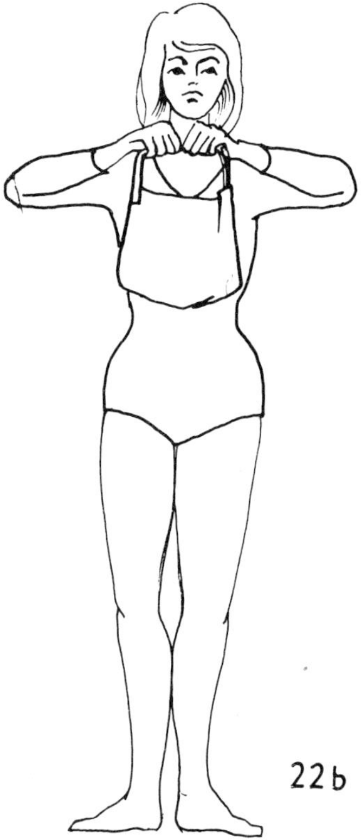

22b

grip on it with the palms facing you and hands the other side of the beam to yourself (Fig. 23a). Take a deep breath and pull yourself up by bending your arms so that you can look over the beam (Fig. 23b). Breathe out as you do so. Lower yourself to the straight-arm position, breathing in as you do so. Your feet are off the floor throughout this exercise, of course.

Do ten repetitions.

2 If you have not got a bar or beam, a useful way of developing the biceps is to stand still and pull a lawn roller or even a heavy mower towards you.

Take an underneath grip on the handle with your hands shoulder width apart (Fig. 24a). Bend your arms to bring the roller or mower towards your feet (Fig. 24b). Walk back until your arms are straight again and repeat the exercise.

Do ten repetitions.

VARIATION ON EXERCISE 7

Take a weight in your right hand. Bend it over your right shoulder and down your back (Fig. 25). Now straighten the arm to raise the weight above your head. Bend it and straighten again.

Do ten repetitions and then change over and do the exercise with the left arm.

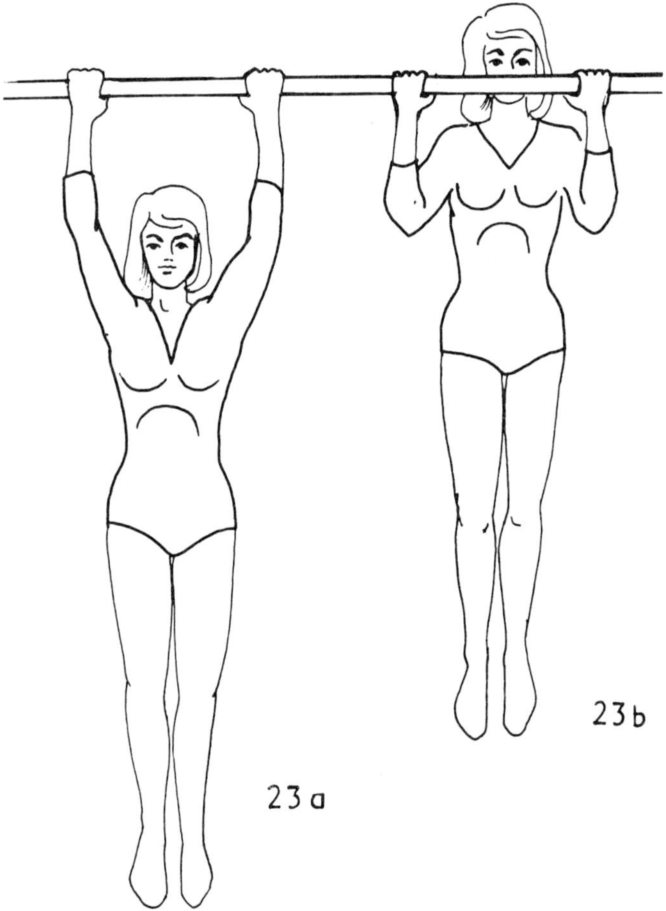

23a 23b

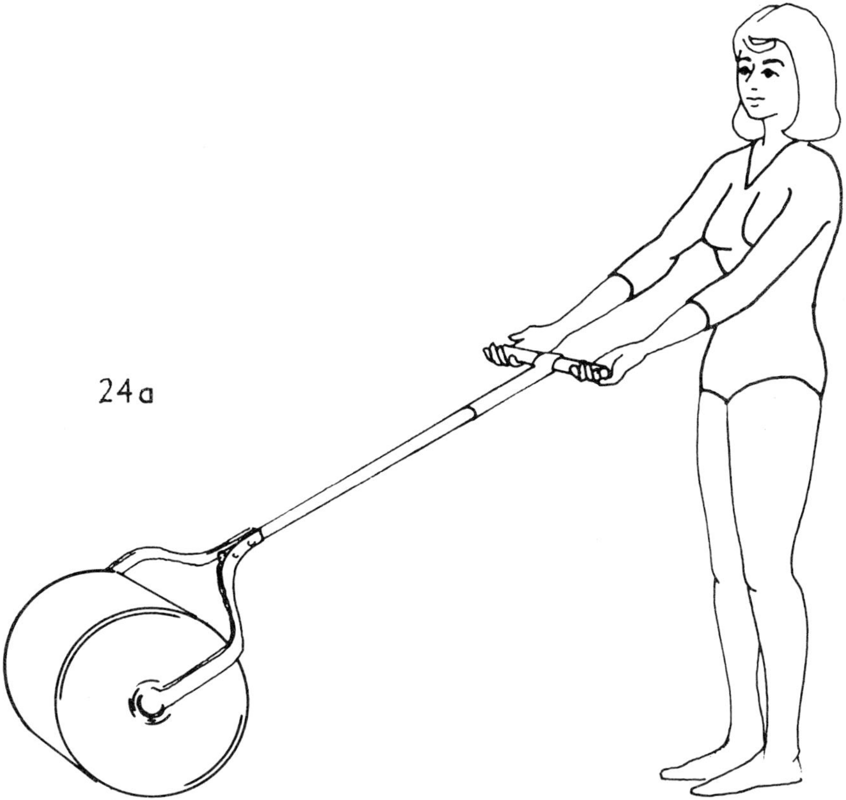

24a

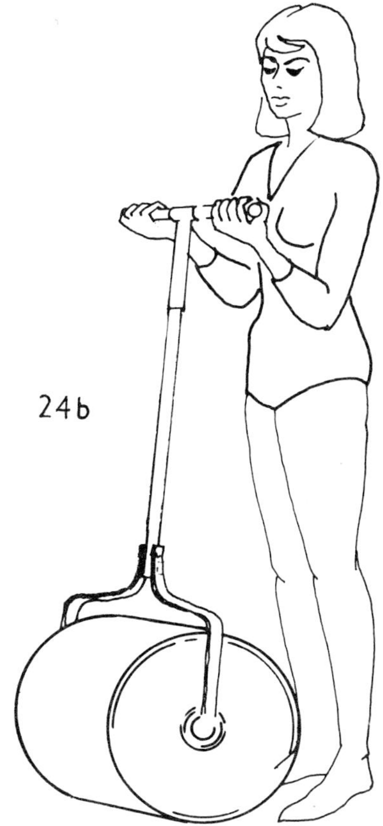

24b

VARIATION ON EXERCISE 8

Hold one arm straight out in front of you, the other arm hanging by your side. Take one corner of a sheet of newspaper in your hand, letting the sheet hang down (Fig. 26). Now gradually gather the sheet up into your hand, crumpling it up into a ball. You may not be able to complete this task at first, but the effort will exercise your wrist and in time you will be strong enough to do so.

Repeat the exercise with the other hand.

VARIATION ON EXERCISE 9

Sit upright on the floor, with the feet wide apart (Fig. 27a). Now alternately touch your left toes with your right hand and then your right toes with your left hand, bending from side to side in a rhythmic, swinging movement (Fig. 27b).

Ten repetitions each side.

VARIATION ON EXERCISE 10

Lie flat on the ground, feet together, arms at your sides (Fig. 28a). Roll to your right, without lifting your

25

26

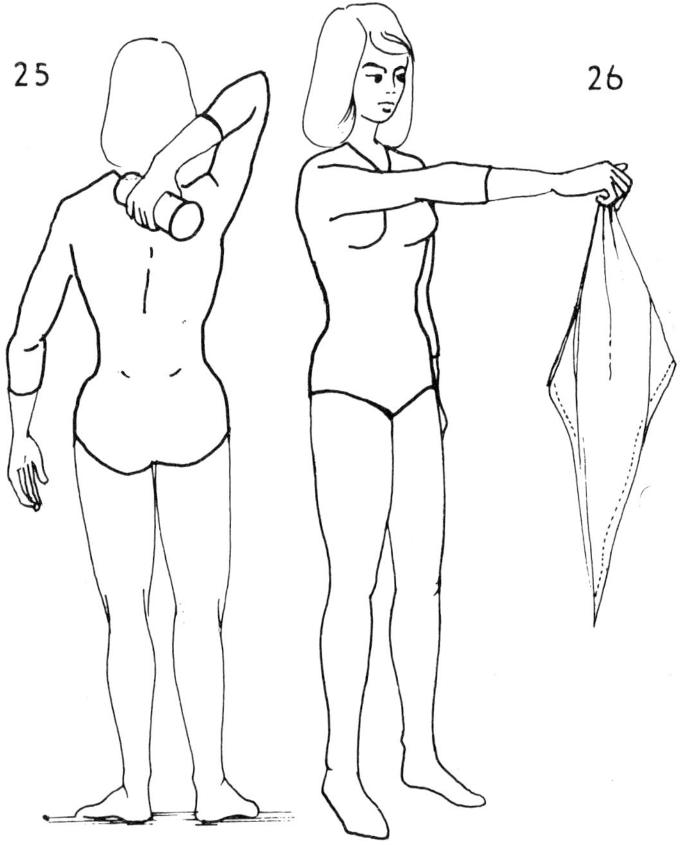

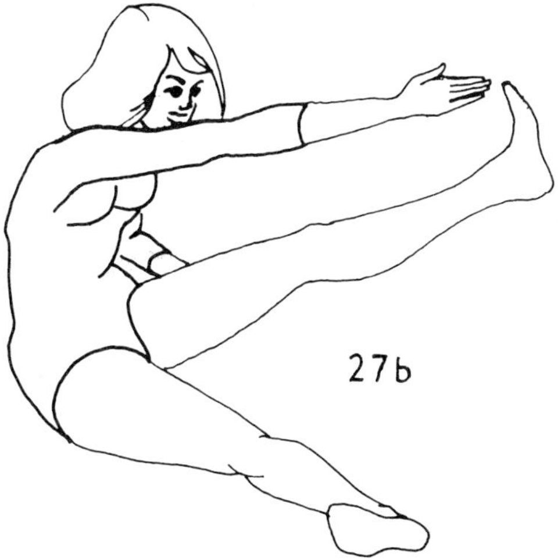

27b

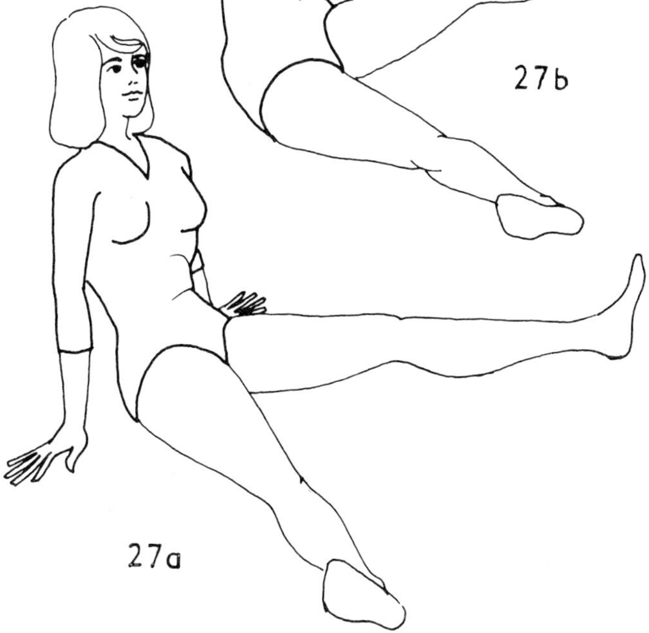

27a

buttocks off the floor, and touch the floor with your left hand at your right side (Fig. 28b). Roll back the other way to your left and touch the floor with your right hand at your left side.

Do ten repetitions with each hand.

VARIATIONS ON EXERCISE 11

1 Lie flat on the floor with hands clasped behind your head (Fig. 29a). Tuck your feet under something to hold them down and then sit up, pulling the head as far down towards your toes as possible with your hands. Breathe out as you do so (Fig. 29b). Lower yourself back to the floor, breathing in as you do so. Control your movement so that you come up as slowly as possible and lower back down slowly. Do not simply flop down.

Do ten repetitions.

2 Lie in the same position as at the beginning of the last exercise (Fig. 29a). Sit up and twist your trunk so that you can touch your knee with the opposite elbow, ie your left knee with your right elbow or vice versa (Fig. 30). Breathe out as you come up.

Go back down and next time you come up touch the other knee with the other elbow, so that you alter-

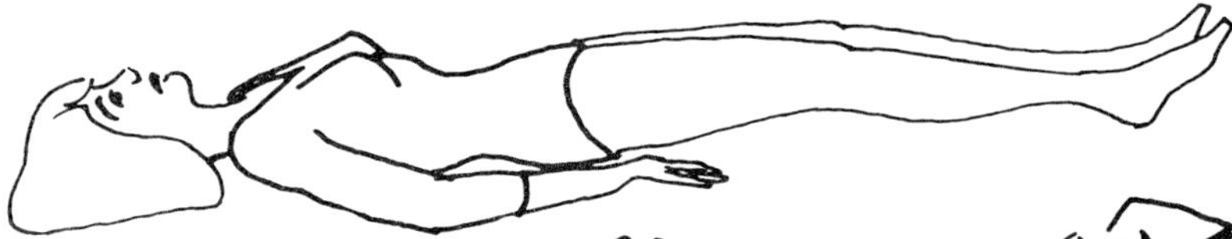

28a

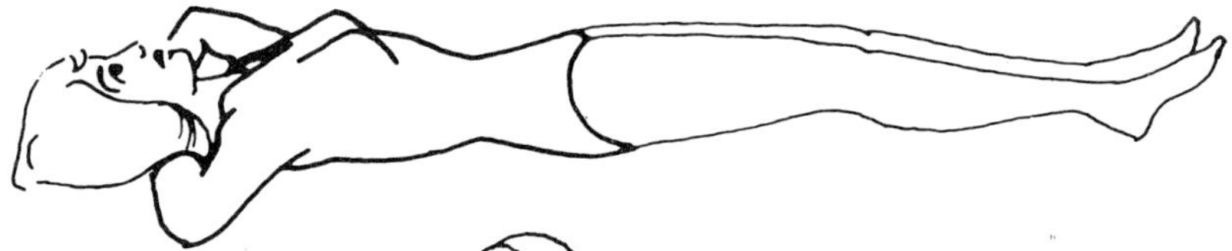

29a

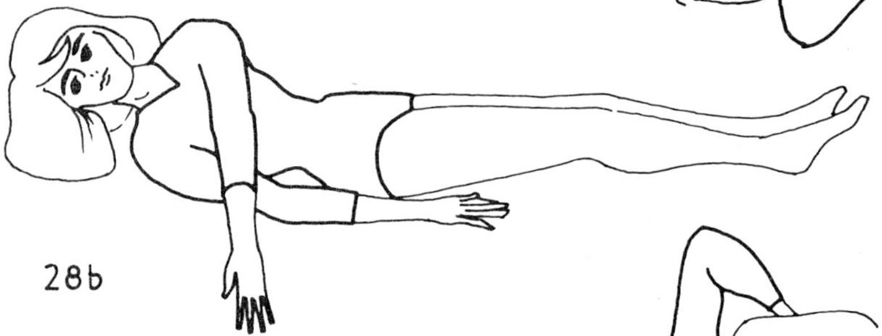

28b

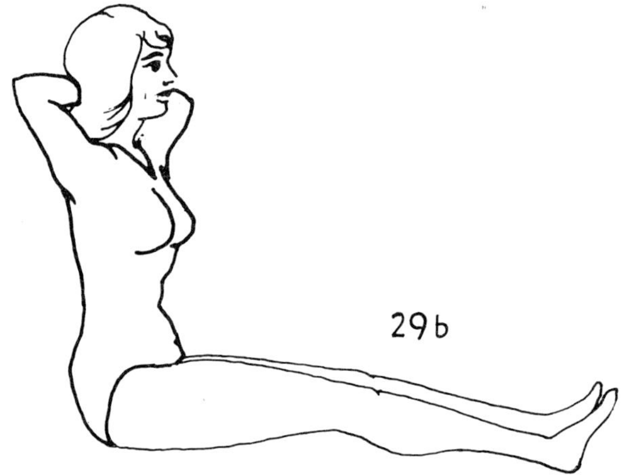

29b

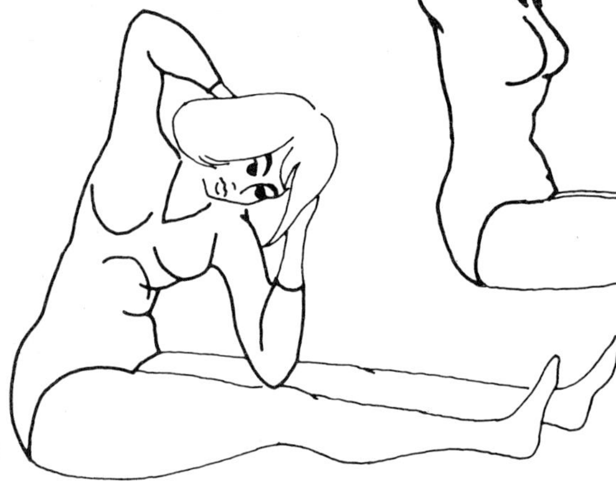

30

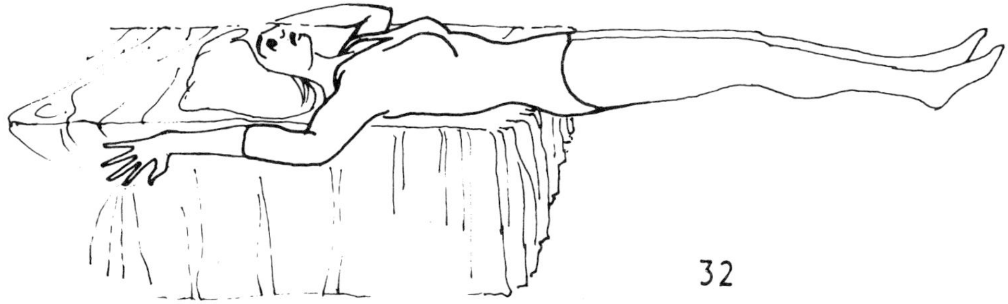

32

31

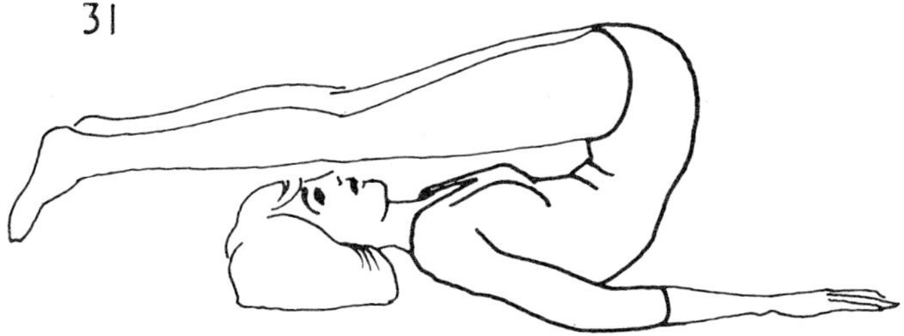

nate the movement. Breathe in as you go down. Try to make it a controlled movement, neither swinging to come up nor flopping back as you go down.

Do ten repetitions altogether.

VARIATIONS ON EXERCISE 12

1 Lie flat on the floor, arms at your sides and feet together as at the beginning of exercise 12 (Fig 14a). This time raise both feet together and take them as far over your head as possible (Fig. 31). Breathe out as you raise the feet and in as you lower them again. Do not put the heels back on the floor, but pause with them an inch or so off the ground and then bring the feet up again.

Do ten repetitions, slowly and with controlled movement.

2 Lie on a bed with your feet off the end. Grasp the sides of the bed with your hands above your head

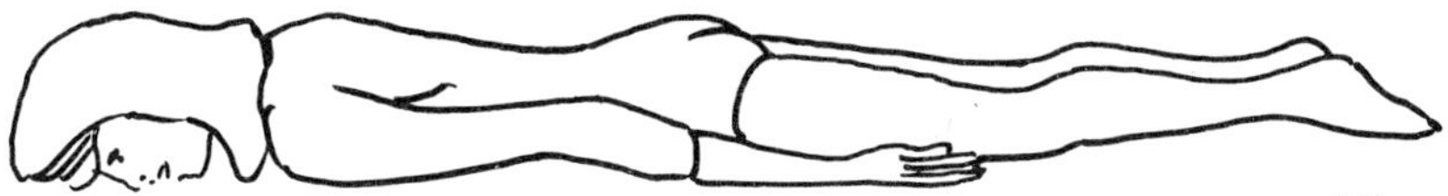

33 a

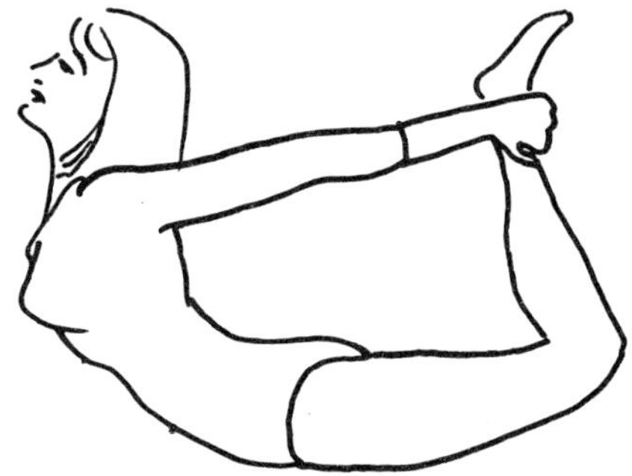

33 b

(Fig. 32). Be as near the end of the bed as you can, so that the abdominal muscles have to support the weight of your legs throughout the exercise. Now raise your legs together slowly, as in the variation you have just done. Breathe out as you raise them. Lower, breathing in, but control the legs so that they stop in the horizontal position and do not droop back down to the floor.

Do ten repetitions.

As a third variation, you can try the alternate leg raise from this position.

VARIATION ON EXERCISE 13

Lie face down, arms at your sides (Fig. 33a). Now raise your feet by bending the knees and take your hands behind you to grasp your feet (Fig. 33b). Lower your feet and hands and then repeat after a brief pause.

Do ten repetitions.

VARIATIONS ON EXERCISE 14

1 Take up the squatting position shown in Fig. 16b. Do ten jumps up into the air, straightening the legs as you come up and bending them as you go back down to the squatting position.

2 Take up the squatting position shown in Fig. 16b. Place the hands on the knees and walk forwards, twice around the room, without straightening up.

VARIATION ON EXERCISE 15

Stand with your feet half on a low step, the heels being off the step. From this position rise on your toes and then lower again.

Do ten repetitions.

VARIATIONS ON EXERCISE 16

These are the same as in variations for exercise 1.

4
Menus to Maintain Fitness

As Chapters 1 and 2 explained, our main requirement of our food is that it should supply our body's basic nutritional needs. If, in addition to this, it does so in a way that is appetising and attractive, we shall benefit further because our digestion will be stimulated and improved.

In this chapter we are going to consider menus for a normal person for a month. I would stress that here we are concerned with the normal reader, not with those wishing to slim or to put on weight. Their special problems are dealt with in Chapters 5 and 6. The menus have been drawn up with some regard for cost, and the foods suggested will be within the ordinary family budget.

Breakfast is such a traditional meal in Britain that the scope for varying it is limited. We can cook eggs in different ways to give some variety; we can vary the cereals and the preserves we eat; we can occasionally have fish; but that is about all the scope there is. None-the-less, this British breakfast with its protein content is much superior to the Continental breakfast of croissants or rolls and butter, since such a breakfast is very stodgy and largely carbohydrate.

After breakfast, each day's menu should contain protein in the form of meat or fish, a variety of vegetables, at least some raw fruit and roughage, and above all a sufficient variety of things to contain all our mineral and vitamin needs. I have therefore suggested one cooked meal and one cold meal containing some form of salad for each day. These meals could be switched from midday to evening as required by the customs of the household. In some families a cooked evening meal is best since it is then that the whole family can be at home; in others the cooked meal is taken in the middle of the day, and the evening meal is a kind of 'high tea'.

Three meals a day should supply our basic needs. The practice of nibbling in between meals not only spoils the appetite but may lead to our nibbling the wrong things, such as sweet biscuits, and so becoming overweight. There is no harm in mid-morning coffee or afternoon tea, but it should be confined to a drink and not made into an extra meal. If we do feel unduly hungry between meals, an apple or other fruit is much better than cake or sweets.

It is not possible within the scope of this book to give specialised diets such as vegetarian or fruitarian ones. There are excellent specialist diet books for people who wish to follow such régimes. We will concern ourselves with a family who will eat whatever is going.

Having said that, however, we must have some regard to individual taste, and recognise that some people are allergic to certain foods. Often in such matters our stomachs know better than our heads and will tell us by rejecting the wrong dishes. If, because of allergy or through personal preference, we decide to omit a certain suggested dish, we must be careful to substitute one which contains the same basic nutrients.

The following menus will take us through a month, giving enough variety to give interest to our meals and to cover all our needs.

WEEK 1

DAY 1, MONDAY

Breakfast Cornflakes, bacon and egg, brown toast (wholemeal bread), honey or marmalade, tea or coffee.

Lunch Cream cheese, pineapple, mixed salad, wholemeal bread and butter, raw apple, tea or coffee.

Dinner Vegetable soup, roast beef, potatoes, greens, gravy, fruit tart with custard or cream, coffee.

DAY 2, TUESDAY

Breakfast Fruit juice, scrambled egg, bread and butter or toast, honey or marmalade, tea or coffee.

Lunch Cold roast beef, mixed salad, pickled onions, bread and butter, raw apple, tea or coffee.

Dinner Minestrone soup, roast chicken, potatoes, carrots, green vegetable, cheese and biscuits, coffee.

DAY 3, WEDNESDAY

Breakfast Cornflakes, poached egg on toast, wholemeal bread, butter, honey or marmalade, tea or coffee.

Lunch Cold chicken, mixed salad, bread and butter, raw orange, tea or coffee.

Dinner Tomato soup, roast lamb with mint sauce, roast potatoes, green vegetable, trifle, custard, coffee.

DAY 4, THURSDAY

Breakfast Grapefruit, kippers, bread and butter, honey or marmalade, tea or coffee.

Lunch Cold roast lamb, mixed salad, bread and butter, raw apple, tea or coffee.

Dinner Mixed grill of bacon, egg, liver, tomatoes and potatoes, yoghurt (or ice cream), coffee.

DAY 5, FRIDAY

Breakfast Cornflakes, bacon and egg, bread and butter or toast, honey or marmalade, tea or coffee.

Lunch Cold ham, mixed salad, bread and butter, orange, tea or coffee.

Dinner White fish with parsley sauce, boiled potatoes, green peas, cheese and biscuits, coffee.

DAY 6, SATURDAY

Breakfast Fruit juice, two boiled eggs, bread and butter or toast, honey or marmalade, tea or coffee.

Lunch Cream cheese, mixed salad, bread and butter, raw apple, tea or coffee.

Dinner Irish stew of potatoes, vegetables, boiled beef, carrots etc, bread, fruit jelly with cream, coffee.

DAY 7, SUNDAY

Breakfast Bran cereal, poached egg, bread and butter or toast, honey or marmalade, tea or coffee.

Lunch Cold ham, mixed salad, bread and butter, orange, tea or coffee.

Dinner Lentil soup, roast beef, greens, roast potatoes, cheese and biscuits, coffee.

WEEK 2

DAY 1, MONDAY

Breakfast Fruit juice, poached haddock, bread and butter, honey or marmalade, tea or coffee.

Lunch Cold beef, salad, bread and butter, raw apple, tea or coffee.

Dinner Asparagus soup, roast chicken, roast potatoes, carrots, greens, onions, cheese, biscuits, coffee.

DAY 2, TUESDAY

Breakfast Cornflakes, bacon and egg, bread and butter, honey or marmalade, tea or coffee.

Lunch Cold chicken, salad, bread and butter, raw apple, tea or coffee.

Dinner Mixed grill of bacon, liver, onions, egg etc, chipped potatoes, fruit salad and cream, coffee.

DAY 3, WEDNESDAY

Breakfast Grapefruit, poached egg on toast, toast with honey or marmalade, tea or coffee.

Lunch Sardine salad, bread and butter, orange, tea or coffee.

Dinner Tomato soup, roast lamb with mint sauce, roast potatoes, greens, cheese and biscuits, coffee.

DAY 4, THURSDAY

Breakfast Cornflakes, boiled eggs, bread and butter, honey or marmalade, tea or coffee.

Lunch Cold lamb, salad, bread and butter, orange, tea or coffee.

Dinner Oxtail soup, ham omelette, French fried potatoes, fruit pie, cream, coffee.

DAY 5, FRIDAY

Breakfast Fruit juice, bacon and egg, bread and butter, honey or marmalade, tea or coffee.

Lunch Cream cheese, salad, bread and butter, raw apple, tea or coffee.

Dinner Grilled halibut steak, parsley sauce, potatoes, peas, fruit salad and cream, coffee.

DAY 6, SATURDAY

Breakfast Cornflakes, scrambled egg on toast, bread and butter, honey or marmalade, tea or coffee.

Lunch Cold ham, salad, bread and butter, raw apple, tea or coffee.

Dinner Irish stew of beef, onions, potatoes, swedes, turnips, carrots etc, bread, cheese and biscuits, coffee.

DAY 7, SUNDAY

Breakfast Bran cereal, bacon and egg, bread and butter, honey or marmalade, tea or coffee.

Lunch Tuna, salad, bread and butter, raw apple, tea or coffee.

Dinner Lentil soup, roast beef, roast potatoes, greens, cheese and biscuits, coffee.

WEEK 3

DAY 1, MONDAY

Breakfast Fruit juice, boiled eggs, bread and butter, honey or marmalade, tea or coffee.

Lunch Cold beef, salad, bread and butter, orange, tea or coffee.

Dinner Mixed grill of bacon, liver, egg, tomatoes etc, boiled potatoes, cheese and biscuits, coffee.

DAY 2, TUESDAY

Breakfast Shredded wheat, bacon and egg, bread and butter, honey or marmalade, tea or coffee.

Lunch Cream cheese, salad, bread and butter, raw apple, tea or coffee.

Dinner Tomato soup, rabbit pie, potatoes, fruit salad and cream, coffee.

DAY 3, WEDNESDAY

Breakfast Fruit juice, kippers, bread and butter, honey or marmalade, tea or coffee.

Lunch Tuna, salad, bread and butter, orange, tea or coffee.

Dinner Minestrone soup, roast chicken, roast potatoes, greens, cheese and biscuits, coffee.

DAY 4, THURSDAY

Breakfast Shredded wheat, scrambled egg, bread and butter, honey or marmalade, tea or coffee.

Lunch Cold chicken, salad, bread and butter, raw apple, tea or coffee.

Dinner Lentil soup, steak and kidney pie, potatoes, peas, trifle, coffee.

DAY 5, FRIDAY

Breakfast Grapefruit, poached egg, bread and butter, honey or marmalade, tea or coffee.

Lunch Cream cheese, salad, bread and butter, orange, tea or coffee.

Dinner Grilled turbot with white sauce, boiled potatoes, peas, fruit pie and cream, coffee.

DAY 6, SATURDAY

Breakfast Fruit juice, bacon and egg, bread and butter, honey or marmalade, tea or coffee.

Lunch Cold ham, salad, bread and butter, raw apple, tea or coffee.

Dinner Irish stew of beef, mixed vegetables, potatoes, etc, cheese and biscuits, coffee.

DAY 7, SUNDAY

Breakfast Bran cereal, boiled eggs, bread and butter, honey or marmalade, tea or coffee.

Lunch Salmon, salad, bread and butter, orange, tea or coffee.

Dinner Vegetable soup, roast beef, roast potatoes, greens, cheese and biscuits, coffee.

WEEK 4

DAY 1, MONDAY

Breakfast Fruit juice, bacon, and egg, bread and butter, honey or marmalade, tea or coffee.

Lunch Cold beef, salad, bread and butter, raw apple, tea or coffee.

Dinner Tomato soup, roast pork and apple sauce, potatoes, peas, cheese and biscuits, coffee.

DAY 2, TUESDAY

Breakfast Cornflakes, boiled egg, bread and butter, honey or marmalade. tea or coffee.

Lunch Cold roast pork, salad, bread and butter, orange, tea or coffee.

Dinner Vegetable soup, roast chicken, potatoes, greens, carrots, cheese and biscuits, coffee.

DAY 3, WEDNESDAY

Breakfast Fruit juice, poached egg, bread and butter, honey or marmalade, tea or coffee.

Lunch Cold chicken, salad, bread and butter, raw apple, tea or coffee.

Dinner Lentil soup, boiled ham and parsley sauce, boiled potatoes, peas, fruit pie and cream, coffee.

DAY 4, THURSDAY

Breakfast Cornflakes, bacon and egg, bread and butter, honey or marmalade, tea or coffee.

Lunch Cold ham, salad, bread and butter, orange, tea or coffee.

Dinner Leek soup, steak and kidney pie, potatoes, peas, cheese and biscuits, coffee.

DAY 5, FRIDAY

Breakfast Grapefruit, scrambled egg, bread and butter, honey or marmalade, tea or coffee.

Lunch Cream cheese, salad, bread and butter, raw apple, tea or coffee.

Dinner Hake, French fried potatoes, bread and butter, fresh fruit salad, cream, coffee.

DAY 6, SATURDAY

Breakfast Fruit juice, bacon and egg, bread and butter, honey or marmalade, tea or coffee.

Lunch Cold ham, salad, bread and butter, raw apple, tea or coffee.

Dinner Oxtail soup, cauliflower cheese, boiled potatoes, apple pie and custard, coffee.

DAY 7, SUNDAY

Breakfast Bran cereal, poached haddock, bread and butter, honey or marmalade, tea or coffee.

Lunch Tuna, salad, bread and butter, orange, coffee or tea.

Dinner Vegetable soup, roast beef, roast potatoes, greens, cheese and biscuits, coffee.

There will, of course, need to be seasonal variations of these meals, and this will be particularly reflected in the salads and to a lesser extent in the vegetables. Vegetables and fruits are obtainable at almost any season of the year, either fresh or frozen, but cost may dictate that we eat fresh vegetables when they are available or when we can grow them in our own gardens. Moreover, freshly gathered vegetables or fruits will certainly be richer in vitamin content.

The salad dishes which form a regular part of our lunches will need to be varied or they will become boring. On some days they can be the traditional mixed salad, consisting of lettuce, cucumber, tomatoes, onions etc. On other days they can take the form of coleslaw, which is made by chopping up cabbage with grated carrot, apple and onion with dates or raisins added. Usually the ready-mixed coleslaw sold in shops has mayonnaise with it, and you can add it to the home-made variety if it is to your taste; but rather less than one gets in the shop product is desirable, and none at all if you are slimming. If neither cabbage nor lettuce is available for salad making, the salad dish can be composed entirely of fruit. Sliced apple with dates is a good combination and goes well with thin slices of Cheddar cheese. Watercress or celery could also take the place of lettuce on occasion.

Under the name of 'greens' for dinner, comes a very wide variety of vegetables. In their season we can have broccoli, cabbage, cauliflower, Brussels sprouts, peas, beans (both runner and broad beans) and spinach. Root vegetables, such as turnips, parsnips, swedes etc, could be served as well or even instead of greens on one or two nights a week.

The fruit pies and fruit salads referred to in the dinner menus can be made from whatever fruit is available. At some seasons strawberries or raspberries will be abundant and fairly cheap, and these are best served fresh. At other times we must fall back on apple pie. When available fresh fruit is always to be preferred to tinned.

As a guide to how we might vary our menus, let us

consider the different seasons in turn.

From December to February old potatoes are available, as are carrots, turnips, swedes, beetroot, leeks, cabbage and celery.

From February to May the old potatoes are generally poor, and tinned ones may be preferred until the new ones start coming in from abroad. With early spring our home-grown new ones will be coming along. Carrots, leeks, cabbages and shallots are available at this time, and citrus fruits will be coming in from Israel.

From June to September, new potatoes become plentiful, and there are fresh peas, beans and cabbages, which some people may grow in their own gardens. The soft fruits come into season at this time, and we shall easily find raspberries, strawberries, blackcurrants, gooseberries, rhubarb, apples, elderberries, whinberries and imported grapes.

In the autumn beetroot, swedes, carrots, parsnips, turnips, sprouts, cabbage, kale, spinach and onions become available. From October to July, watercress is plentiful, as it is grown in heated beds during the winter.

During the winter months it is quite a good idea to have porridge instead of the cornflake type of cereal for breakfast, as it gives us warmth to begin the day. In summer, on the other hand, it is often a good idea to substitute fruit juice for the soup course at dinner. Yoghurt as a sweet is an acquired taste; some people never grow to like it, but for those who do, it undoubtedly has good food value.

Each day I have tried to include some cheese in our menus. Here too we should try to have variety. The cream cheeses and the milder ones such as Cheddar, Cheshire etc, are probably best with salads. The richer ones such as Danish Blue or Stilton are more suitable for the cheese and biscuit course that follows the main dish at dinner.

There is, of course, no reason why we should not have wine with our dinner if we like it, as a little aids digestion; but for our health's sake we should be moderate in our drinking habits. At most meals I have specified tea or coffee since these are traditional British beverages, but water is a good substitute for either, and fruit cordials may be preferred by some people. There is not a lot of nutrition in tea or coffee. They are mild stimulants and so comfort us, but their food value is largely confined to their milk, sugar and water content.

5
How to lose those Extra Pounds

Years ago it was considered quite natural to be overweight, particularly in middle age, and no one worried too much about the state. Today, however, we know that this condition is bad for us, and most sufferers want to do something about it.

WHAT IS BEING OVERWEIGHT?

Being overweight means simply having an excess of body fat. We know that essentially our bodies consist of a skeleton of bones covered with muscle and fat and containing various internal organs, kept going by a blood supply. Some fat is essential to our well-being. The fat under our skin insulates our body and keeps us warm. Other areas of fat act as cushions, not only in such places as the soles of our feet and our buttocks, but also around the heart, the lungs and the intestines. Fat keeps our muscles separate, and fat in the joints makes them move easily. We cannot live without fat, but it is when it becomes excessive that the dangers of obesity arise.

HOW DO WE TELL WHEN IT IS EXCESSIVE?

Consult the tables given in Chapter 2. If you have consciously set out to develop your physique you may be above average in weight and still not have excess fat. If you suffer from some illness, such as water retention, you may be over the weight suggested for your height and still not have excess fat. But if you are a normal person then anything much over the figures quoted means that you are overweight and must lose some fat.

HOW DO WE BECOME OVERWEIGHT?

There are two kinds of obesity known as exogenous obesity and endogenous obesity. The first arises through overeating, the second through the body not coping properly with the food we do eat.

Endogenous obesity arises from improper functioning of one or more of the internal glands, such as the thyroid, the pituitary, the ovaries or the testicles, or the suprarenal glands. All these cases require medical attention and if our weight problem is of the endogenous variety, we must consult a doctor. It is no good trying to treat ourselves.

Exogenous obesity is by far the most common kind and it is the one in which we can help ourselves. Overeating arises partly from the higher living standards we enjoy today. We could not overeat during the last war because we did not get enough food to do so; and in some ways we were healthier for our deprivation.

Eating between meals, especially such things as sweets and biscuits, will contribute to a weight problem. The housewife is at particular risk. A woman has a greater storage capacity for fat than a man because she is physically adapted to holding greater reserves in preparation for the bearing and feeding of children. When she has had children she usually gives up outside work at least for a few years, in order to stay at home and look after them. It is during this time that the tendency to nibble between meals starts.

Cooks usually taste a little of what they are cooking to see if the dish is coming up to their expectations or if it is done. Mothers whose children refuse food will sometimes clear the plate themselves to avoid waste, not realising that by doing so they are having an extra portion. Women at home often have friends dropping in for morning coffee or afternoon tea, usually served with biscuits or cakes. Taking all these things together, it will be easily understood that the housewife can overeat without knowing that she is doing so.

Middle-aged people are another group who are prone to becoming overweight. They tend to have given up or to have cut down on their physical activities. They believe that sports are for the young and not for them. Greater prosperity means that they ride to work in a car instead of walking or cycling. Simultaneously with this cutting down of physical activity, they are entering a period of life when their metabolic rate (the rate at which we use up the food we eat) is slowing down. In the young, the metabolic rate will alter to correct dietary errors to a certain extent, but this will not happen with an older person. If the middle-aged man cuts down exercise without altering his diet, he will become overweight as a result.

Even children suffer from obesity today. Statistics have shown that about 3 per cent must be regarded as over the desirable weight. This is a small percentage as compared with the adult population, where the figure is 50 per cent, but fatness is even more serious in children, and usually the fat child will become a fat adult.

WHY WORRY ABOUT IT?

'Worry' is perhaps hardly the word to use. We will not help anything by worrying. But concerned we should be, because being overweight can injure our health and shorten our lives. It has been estimated that each pound of excess weight we carry will take one month off our lives. Our bodies are only designed to carry a certain weight. Any excess puts a strain on all the organs.

When you go shopping and come home with a heavy basket in each hand, you are carrying twenty to thirty pounds in weight. You know what it feels like. You are slower getting on the bus; you puff when you climb a hill; your arms ache. You know that you are carrying those twenty or thirty pounds. But if you are twenty or thirty pounds overweight, you are putting this kind of extra strain on your body all the time.

You will be more susceptible to coronary and renal troubles, to cirrhosis of the liver, to gallstones, or to diabetes mellitus, to mention only a few of the ills that attack overweight men and women. Your slowness of movement will tend to increase your problem since you will not burn up as much fat getting around. You will quickly get out of breath. If your obesity becomes unsightly you may hesitate to take part in social life, and once you start sitting at home watching television instead of going out and about you will make your problem still worse by not taking any exercise at all.

The danger, then, is that you will become a compulsive eater to make up for your lack of other interests. Obesity must be regarded as a disease. Like other diseases, it will be progressive if not treated.

Children suffer perhaps more than adults from the physical and psychological ills of fatness. Fat children are often an object of fun to their fellows, and children can be terribly cruel to each other. Because fat boys and girls are not very good at games, they become unpopular. They may even be lonely, and then they will tend to take refuge in the only pleasure they know – eating sweets to comfort themselves – and so make their fatness worse.

WHAT CAN WE DO ABOUT BEING OVERWEIGHT?

In the case of a child, consult a doctor first. Most cases of fatness in children are either hereditary or glandular. It is essential that medical advice be sought.

Part of the cure may be diet. If the doctor recommends this, there is a lot we can do to help the child to keep to the diet. Do not serve his favourite dish to other members of the family when it is forbidden to your child. Try to adjust the whole family diet. Cutting down on the carbohydrates and stepping up the proteins will help you all. Make it a family rule not to have sweets in the house. If the family want something between meals or if you want to give the child a treat, offer fruit instead of sweets. Keep any child on a diet active and interested. Help him to start new hobbies or to find new friends. Both activities often go together. Anything you can do on the above lines will help the cure.

In the case of an overweight adult with an endogenous condition, medical help will be needed in the same way as for a child. If, however, our condition is simply due to overeating we can help ourselves.

The general routine of exercises given in chapter 3 will tone up our body and give us some regular, physical activity. Following that routine should, therefore, be of help. Adjusting our diet should do the rest.

There are various diets designed to lose weight. All of them have their devotees, however faddish some of them may be. The first diet to be published was Banting's in 1863, so dieting is not a modern craze.

Obesity arises from the number of calories we put into our bodies in the form of food being greater than the number we expend in the form of energy. To maintain balance our intake must equal our output; to reduce our weight our intake must be lower than our output, so that some of our reserves will be used up. To lose 1lb of weight in a week, there needs to be a calorie deficit of 500 per day. You could get rid of this number by a two-hour brisk walk. You could get rid of it by not taking sugar in your tea. Most people find that extra exercise on its own is too exhausting a way of losing the calories. They combine extra exercise with some form of dieting.

The simplest diet is to eat smaller portions of everything. This is a system that has its adherents. The argument against it is that it assumes you are already eating all your nutrients in excess and that the excesses are in the same proportion. Even if your diet is well balanced, by cutting every item to the same extent you run the risk of falling below the minimum requirement in some essential nutrient (*see* Chapter 1).

The safest and perhaps the commonest diet is the low carbohydrate diet. In this you eat the same quantities of protein and fat as you usually do, but you reduce your carbohydrate intake. Very simply, it is largely a case of cutting out sugar in drinks and reducing the amount of bread and the number of potatoes you eat.

If your daily requirement of calories is assessed at 2,500, you can very well cut it to 1,500, and this would produce a weight loss of 1½–2lb a week. The loss will not necessarily be regular, as some people respond differently to diet than others. In one person dieting may produce results in spasms with a big loss one week and very little the next. Do not weigh yourself every day or every week, therefore, as you may feel you are not succeeding. A bad week would discourage you, and would not necessarily mean that your diet was wrong. You should give any diet at least a month's trial. After the first month by all means weigh weekly. The average loss of 1½–2lb a week would be seen over a period of two or three months.

To assist you in cutting your carbohydrate intake there are many slimming foods on the market. There are low-calorie fruit drinks and low-calorie mayonnaise; the slimming breads, though not quite as satisfying to the taste, give 35 calories to the slice as compared with 52 from ordinary bread; and probably of most help to you will be the sweeteners you can use instead of sugar. There are several brands, and they can be used in puddings and cakes as well as in drinks, thus saving extra calories all the time. If you drink six cups of tea or coffee a day, you could save 450 calories by simply putting in a sweetener instead of sugar. This would be almost half of the thousand you are trying to save.

In this chapter I will give specimen menus for a month based on a daily intake of just over 1,500 calories per day. This is not at all rigorous. You could follow it for six months or a year, and at the end of that time you would certainly see results. If you want a quicker solution to your problem you must think of cutting to 1,000 calories per day, but bear in mind that crash diets like this can only be followed for a very limited time, and their very severity tends to put people off. It is better to aim at a more modest weight reduction over a longer period. This is possible on the 1,500 calorie diet I have outlined, and you will be able to keep it up.

Since tastes in food differ, and there is no reason why you should not eat the dishes you prefer, I have indicated alternative dishes with the same calorie value so that you can substitute them. I have also shown the calorie value of each item, because it is essential to your slimming programme that you think about counting calories for yourself.

It is best to have a good breakfast and to have your other meals at the normal times. You need not cut out mid-morning coffee or afternoon tea when following this diet, providing that you use sweeteners in the drinks and not sugar and providing that you do not accompany the drinks with cakes or biscuits. You must remember that two teaspoonfuls of sugar in your teacup would add 75 calories to your total for that day. You would have to give up a slice of bread and butter to make up for a lapse like that, and this is how you must begin to think of your diet, counting calories and balancing one extra treat against a self-restraint in another direction.

You will see that the slimming menus I give in this chapter do not differ drastically from the menus I have given in Chapter 4. The main difference between the slimmer and the ordinary person is that the slimmer has to study the quantities of food he is eating, and has to cut down on sugar, potatoes and bread. It is, therefore, possible for the housewife to slim herself whilst serving the ordinary non-slimming meals given in Chapter 4 to the rest of her family. The convenience of this will be appreciated by anyone who has tried to cook for a family. The menus in this chapter are essentially those of Chapter 4 with the slight variations needed to enable you to slim.

If, when trying this diet, you still feel hungry, do not despair and give up. There are foods on which you can fill up without disturbing your diet. Eat as much kidney beans, runner beans, spinach, asparagus, tomatoes, cauliflower, broccoli, sprouts, cabbage, lettuce, cucumber, radish, onions, watercress or celery as you desire.

I can hear the critics crying 'rabbit food', but these items do fill the hole. If you feel, after trying honestly to follow this diet, that you cannot exist on 1,500 calories per day, owing perhaps to especially strenuous work or some similar circumstance, then vary it by increasing your protein intake not your carbohydrate. Eat more meat, fish and eggs.

Do not drop below 1,500 calories per day for any lengthy period unless on medical advice, as such self-imposed restriction could be dangerous.

WEEK 1

DAY 1, MONDAY

	Number of calories
Breakfast	
½ grapefruit with no sugar	12
1 boiled egg	92
1 large slice brown bread	119
Tea with sweetener	—
½pt (284ml) milk for the day	190
1½oz (42g) butter for the day	339
Lunch	
2 oz (56g) cottage cheese	66
1 slice bread	119
4oz (113g) lettuce	12
1oz (28g) cucumber	2
2oz (56g) tomatoes	6
1 eating apple (4oz size)	40
Tea or coffee with sweetener	—
Dinner	
3oz (85g) beef	210
3oz (85g) potatoes	51
3oz (85g) cabbage	36
3oz (85g) stewed apples	24
1oz (28g) ice cream	56
Tea or coffee with sweetener	—
Total calories for day 1	1,374

DAY 2, TUESDAY

Breakfast	
2fl oz unsweetened orange juice	45
Scrambled egg	92
1 large slice bread	119
1½oz (42g) butter for the day	339
½pt milk for the day	190
Tea with sweetener	—
Lunch	
3oz (85g) cold roast beef	220
1 slice bread	119
Mixed salad, details as yesterday	20
4oz (113g) eating apple	40
Tea or coffee with sweetener	—
Dinner	
3oz (85g) roast chicken	150
3oz (85g) potatoes	51
3oz (85g) carrots	16
Banana Split (made with ice cream, banana and a sauce of strawberry jam)	180
Coffee with sweetener	—
Total calories for day 2	1,581

DAY 3, WEDNESDAY

Breakfast

½ grapefruit without sugar	12
poached egg on 1 slice of toast	211
1½oz (42g) of butter for the day	339
½pt of milk for day	190
Tea with sweetener	—

Lunch

3oz (85g) cold chicken	150
Salad, mixed as yesterday	20
1 slice bread	119
Raw orange	24
Tea or coffee with sweetener	—

Dinner

3oz (85g) roast lamb	207
3oz (85g) potatoes	51
3oz (85g) greens	36
Mandarin oranges in ice cream	177
Coffee with sweetener	—

Total calories for day 3	1,536

DAY 4, THURSDAY

Breakfast

2oz (56g) unsweetened fruit juice	45
3oz (85g) kippers	114
1 slice bread	119
1½oz (42g) butter for the day	339
½pt milk for day	190
Tea or coffee with sweetener	—

Lunch

3oz (85g) cold lamb	207
Salad as before	20
1 slice bread	119
Raw orange	24
Tea or coffee with sweetener	—

Dinner

2oz (56g) fried bacon	266
2oz (56g) fried tomatoes	6
3oz (85g) potatoes	51
Roast apple	40
Coffee with sweetener	—

Total calories for Day 4	1,540

DAY 5, FRIDAY

Breakfast

½ grapefruit without sugar	12
Poached egg on 1 slice bread or toast	211
1½oz (42g) of butter for the day	339
½pt of milk for the day	190
Tea with sweetener	—

Lunch

3oz (85g) ham	291
Salad as before	20
1 slice bread	119
Raw apple	40
Tea or coffee with sweetener	—

Dinner

4oz (113g) cod	53
Parsley sauce	3
3oz (85g) potatoes	51
Peach Melba (peaches and ice cream)	185
Coffee with sweetener	—

Total calories for day 5	1,514

DAY 6, SATURDAY

Breakfast

2fl oz (56g) unsweetened fruit juice	45
Boiled egg	92
1 slice bread or toast	119
1½oz (42g) of butter for the whole day	339
½pt of milk for the day	190
Tea with sweetener	—

Lunch

2oz (56g) cheese	212
Salad as before	20
1 slice bread	119
Orange	24
Tea or coffee with sweetener	—

Dinner

Stew consisting of:	
2oz (56g) boiled beef	186
2oz (56g) potatoes	34
Mixed vegetables (onions, carrots etc)	20
Jelly with cream	135
Coffee with sweetener	—

Total calories for day 6	1,535

DAY 7, SUNDAY

Breakfast

½ grapefruit without sugar	12
Scrambled egg	92
1 slice bread	119
1½oz (42g) butter for the day	339
½pt milk for the day	190
Tea with sweetener	—

Lunch

3oz (85g) cold ham	291
Salad as before	20
1 slice bread	119
Raw apple (4oz size)	40
Tea or coffee with sweetener	—

Dinner

3oz (85g) roast beef	210
3oz (85g) potatoes	51
3oz (85g) greens	36
Orange	24
Coffee with sweetener	—

Total calories for day 7	1,543

WEEK 2

DAY 1, MONDAY

Breakfast

2fl oz (56g) unsweetened fruit juice	45
4oz (113g) poached haddock (smoked)	50
1 slice bread	119
1½oz (42g) butter for the day	339
½pt milk for the day	190
Tea with sweetener	—

Lunch

3oz (85g) cold beef	210
Salad	20
1 slice bread	119
Orange	24
Tea or coffee with sweetener	—

Dinner

A hot-pot consisting of:	
3oz (85g) roast chicken	150
2oz (56g) cabbage	24
1 carrot	6
1 onion	7
Raw pear	18
Coffee with sweetener	—

Total calories for day 1	1,321

DAY 2, TUESDAY

Breakfast	
½ grapefruit	12
Boiled egg	92
1 slice bread	119
1½oz (42g) butter for the day	339
½pt milk for the day	190
Tea with sweetener	—
Lunch	
3oz (85g) cold chicken	150
Salad	20
1 slice bread	119
Raw apple	40
Tea or coffee with sweetener	—
Dinner	
4oz (113g) grilled liver	164
Fried onion	7
3oz (85g) French fried potatoes	200
4oz (113g) grapes	56
Coffee with sweetener	—
Total calories for Day 2	1,508

DAY 3, WEDNESDAY

Breakfast	
2fl oz (56g) unsweetened fruit juice	45
Poached egg	92
1 slice bread	119
1½oz (42g) butter for the day	339
½pt milk for the day	190
Tea with sweetener	—
Lunch	
2oz (56g) sardines (drain off oil)	168
Salad	20
1 slice bread	119
Orange	24
Tea or coffee with sweetener	—
Dinner	
3oz (85g) roast lamb	207
3oz (85g) roast potatoes	51
3oz (85g) greens	36
Raw apple	40
Coffee with sweetener	—
Total calories for day 3	1,450

DAY 4, THURSDAY

Breakfast	
½ grapefruit	12
Boiled egg	92
1 slice bread	119
1½oz (42g) butter for the day	339
½pt of milk for the day	190
Tea with sweetener	—
Lunch	
3oz (85g) cold lamb	207
Salad	20
1 slice bread	119
Apple	40
Tea or coffee with sweetener	—
Dinner	
Omelette made with 2 eggs and 1oz (28g) ham	279
2oz (56g) ice cream	112
Coffee with sweetener	—
Total calories for day 4	1,529

DAY 5, FRIDAY

Breakfast	
2fl oz (56g) unsweetened fruit juice	45
Fried egg	92
1 slice toast	119
1½oz (42g) butter for the day	339
½pt milk for the day	190
Tea with sweetener	—
Lunch	
2oz (56g) cottage cheese	66
Salad	20
1 slice bread	119
Orange	24
Tea or coffee with sweetener	—
Dinner	
4oz (113g) grilled halibut steak	72
Parsley sauce	7
3oz (85g) boiled potatoes	51
3oz (85g) green peas	21
Banana Split (banana and ice cream)	180
Coffee with sweetener	—
Total calories for day 5	1,345

DAY 6, SATURDAY

Breakfast	
½ grapefruit	12
Scrambled egg	92
1 slice toast	119
1½oz (42g) butter for the day	339
½pt milk for the day	190
Tea with sweetener	—
Lunch	
3oz (85g) cold ham	291
Salad	20
1 slice bread	119
Raw apple	40
Tea or coffee with sweetener	—
Dinner	
Stew made with:	
2oz (56g) boiled beef	186
2oz (56g) potatoes	34
Onions, carrots etc	20
Orange	24
Coffee with sweetener	—
Total calories for day 6	1,486

DAY 7, SUNDAY

Breakfast	
2fl oz (56g) unsweetened fruit juice	45
Boiled egg	92
1 slice bread	119
1½oz (42g) butter for the day	339
½pt milk for the day	190
Tea with sweetener	—
Lunch	
3oz (85g) tinned tuna (drain off oil)	177
Salad	20
1 slice bread	119
Orange	24
Tea or coffee with sweetener	—
Dinner	
3oz (85g) roast beef	210
3oz (85g) potatoes	51
3oz (85g) greens	36
Raw apple	40
Coffee with sweetener	—
Total calories for day 7	1,462

DAY 1, MONDAY

Breakfast

½ grapefruit	12
Boiled egg	92
1 slice bread	119
1½oz (42g) butter for the day	339
½pt milk for the day	190
Tea with sweetener	—

Lunch

3oz (85g) cold beef	210
Salad	20
1 slice bread	119
Apple	40
Tea or coffee with sweetener	—

Dinner

4oz (113g) grilled liver with onions and tomatoes	180
3oz (85g) boiled potatoes	51
1oz (28g) Cheddar cheese	120
Crispbread (2 pieces)	66
Coffee with sweetener	—

Total calories for day 1 1,558

DAY 2, TUESDAY

Breakfast

2fl oz (56g) unsweetened fruit juice	45
Fried egg	92
1 slice bread	119
1½oz (42g) butter for the day	339
½pt milk for the day	190
Tea with sweetener	—

Lunch

2oz (56g) cottage cheese	66
Salad	20
1 slice bread	119
Orange	24
Tea or coffee with sweetener	—

Dinner

Rabbit pie (3oz (85g) rabbit and	96
other ingredients)	100
4oz (113g) fruit salad with	88
1oz cream	62
Coffee with sweetener	—

Total calories for day 2 1,360

DAY 3, WEDNESDAY

Breakfast

½ grapefruit	12
3oz (85g) kippers grilled	114
1 slice bread	119
1½oz (42g) butter for the day	339
½pt milk for the day	190
Tea with sweetener	—

Lunch

3oz (85g) tuna (drain off oil)	177
Salad	20
1 slice bread	119
Apple	40
Tea or coffee with sweetener	—

Dinner

3oz (85g) roast chicken	150
3oz (85g) potatoes	51
3oz (85g) greens	36
1oz (28g) Cheddar cheese	120
2 crispbreads	66
Coffee with sweetener	—

Total calories for day 3	1,553

DAY 4, THURSDAY

Breakfast

2fl oz (56g) unsweetened fruit juice	45
Scrambled egg	92
1 slice bread	119
1½oz (42g) butter for the day	339
½pt milk for the day	190
Tea with sweetener	—

Lunch

3oz (85g) cold chicken	150
Salad	20
1 slice bread	119
Orange	24
Tea or coffee with sweetener	—

Dinner

3oz (85g) steak and kidney pie	200
3oz (85g) boiled potatoes	51
Trifle	100
Coffee with sweetener	—

Total calories for day 4	1,449

DAY 5, FRIDAY

Breakfast	
½ grapefruit	12
Poached egg	92
1 slice toast	119
1½oz (42g) butter for the day	339
½pt milk for the day	190
Tea with sweetener	—
Lunch	
2oz (56g) cottage cheese	66
Salad	20
1 slice bread	119
Apple	40
Tea or coffee with sweetener	—
Dinner	
4oz (113g) grilled turbot	72
3oz (85g) boiled potatoes	51
3oz (85g) green peas	21
Small fruit pie	195
Coffee with sweetener	—
Total calories for day 5	1,336

DAY 6, SATURDAY

Breakfast	
2fl oz (56g) unsweetened fruit juice	45
Boiled egg	92
1 slice bread	119
1½oz (42g) butter for the day	339
½pt milk for the day	190
Tea with sweetener	—
Lunch	
3oz (85g) cold ham	291
Salad	20
1 slice bread	119
Orange	24
Tea or coffee with sweetener	—
Dinner	
Irish stew made of:	
2oz (56g) boiled beef,	
2oz (56g) potatoes, onion, carrots etc	240
Raw apple	40
Coffee with sweetener	—
Total calories for day 6	1,519

DAY 7, SUNDAY

Breakfast

½ grapefruit	12
Boiled egg	92
1 slice bread	119
1½oz (42g) butter for the day	339
½pt milk for the day	190
Tea with sweetener	—

Lunch

3oz (85g) tinned salmon (drain off oil)	105
Salad	20
1 slice bread	119
Apple	40
Tea or coffee with sweetener	—

Dinner

3oz (85g) roast beef	210
3oz (85g) roast potatoes	51
3oz (85g) greens	36
1oz (28g) Cheddar cheese	120
2 crispbreads	66
Coffee with sweetener	—

Total calories for day 7	1,519

WEEK 4

DAY 1, MONDAY

Breakfast

2fl oz (56g) unsweetened fruit juice	45
Fried egg	92
1 slice bread	119
1½oz (42g) butter for the day	339
½pt milk for the day	190
Tea with sweetener	—

Lunch

3oz (85g) cold beef	210
Salad	20
1 slice bread	119
Orange	24
Tea or coffee with sweetener	—

Dinner

3oz (85g) roast pork	219
Apple sauce	20
3oz (85g) boiled potatoes	51
3oz (85g) fresh green peas	21
Apple	40
Coffee with sweetener	—

Total calories for day 1	1,509

DAY 2, TUESDAY

Breakfast	
½ grapefruit	12
Boiled egg	92
1 slice bread	119
1½oz (42g) butter for the day	339
½pt milk for the day	190
Tea or coffee with sweetener	—
Lunch	
3oz (85g) cold roast pork (shoulder)	219
Salad	20
1 slice bread	119
Apple	40
Tea or coffee with sweetener	—
Dinner	
3oz (85g) roast chicken	150
3oz (85g) potatoes	51
3oz (85g) greens	36
1oz (28g) Cheddar cheese	120
2 crispbreads	66
Coffee with sweetener	—
Total calories for day 2	1,573

DAY 3, WEDNESDAY

Breakfast	
2fl oz (56g) unsweetened fruit juice	45
Poached egg	92
1 slice toast	119
1½oz (42g) butter for the day	339
½pt milk for the day	190
Tea with sweetener	—
Lunch	
3oz (85g) cold chicken	150
Salad	20
1 slice bread	119
Orange	24
Tea or coffee with sweetener	—
Dinner	
3oz (85g) boiled ham	291
3oz (85g) potatoes	51
3oz (85g) green peas	21
Raw apple	40
Coffee with sweetener	—
Total calories for day 3	1,501

DAY 4, THURSDAY

Breakfast	
½ grapefruit	12
Fried egg	92
1 slice bread	119
1½oz (42g) butter for the day	339
½pt milk for the day	190
Tea with sweetener	—
Lunch	
3oz (85g) cold ham	291
Salad	20
1 slice bread	119
Apple	40
Tea or coffee with sweetener	—
Dinner	
3oz (85g) steak and kidney pie	200
3oz (85g) potatoes	51
Orange	24
Coffee with sweetener	—
Total calories for day 4	1,497

DAY 5, FRIDAY

Breakfast	
2fl oz (56g) unsweetened fruit juice	45
Scrambled egg	92
1 slice toast	119
1½oz (42g) butter for the day	339
½pt milk for the day	190
Tea with sweetener	—
Lunch	
2oz (56g) cottage cheese	66
Salad	20
1 slice bread	119
Orange	24
Tea or coffee with sweetener	—
Dinner	
4oz (113g) boiled hake	75
3oz (85g) French fried potatoes	200
4oz (113g) fruit salad with	88
1oz (28g) cream	62
Coffee with sweetener	—
Total calories for day 5	1,439

DAY 6, SATURDAY

Breakfast	
½ grapefruit	12
Fried egg	92
1 slice bread	119
1½oz (42g) butter for the day	339
½pt milk for the day	190
Tea with sweetener	—
Lunch	
3oz (85g) cold ham	291
Salad	20
1 slice bread	119
Apple	40
Tea or coffee with sweetener	—
Dinner	
Cauliflower cheese:	
2oz (56g) cheese	272
8oz (226g) cauliflower	
2oz (56g) potatoes	34
Orange	24
Coffee with sweetener	—
Total calories for day 6	1,552

DAY 7, SUNDAY

Breakfast	
2fl oz (56g) unsweetened fruit juice	45
4oz (113g) poached smoked haddock	50
1 slice bread	119
1½oz (42g) butter for the day	339
½pt milk for the day	190
Tea with sweetener	—
Lunch	
3oz (85g) tuna (drain off oil)	177
Salad	20
1 slice bread	119
Orange	24
Tea or coffee with sweetener	—
Dinner	
3oz (85g) roast beef	210
3oz (85g) boiled potatoes	51
3oz (85g) greens	36
2oz (56g) Cheddar cheese	120
2 crispbreads	66
Coffee with sweetener	—
Total calories for day 7	1,566

You may not like all the foods suggested in this diet, alternative main dishes and sweets with their calorie values are listed so that you can work out for yourselves how to substitute. We are not concerned with a small calorie variation of say up to 50 calories in a day, but if the dish you substitute is going to increase your calories by more than that figure, you must leave out some other item to compensate, or have a smaller helping.

Meat dishes	*Calorie values (per oz (28g))*
Gammon	92
Middle-cut bacon	133
Roast beef	73
Sirloin steak	68
Chicken	54
Turkey	56
Duckling	136
Mutton (leg)	59
Mutton chop	91
Leg of pork	71
Veal	32
Beef sausages	75
Pork sausages	101
Kidney	36
Liver	41
Corned beef	66
Ham	97
Luncheon meat	95

Fish dishes	
Filleted cod	20
Salt cod	15
Filleted haddock	20
Smoked haddock	12
Hake	19
Halibut	18
Herrings	38
Mackerel	24
Pilchards (tinned) in tomato sauce	63
Plaice	12
Salmon (tinned)	39
Sardines (tinned) in oil	84
Tuna (tinned)	59

Cheeses	
Camembert	88
Cheddar	120
Cheshire	110

Cottage cheese	33
Danish blue	103
Edam (the lowest apart from cottage cheese)	88
Gorgonzola	112
Processed	106
Stilton	135
Wensleydale	115

Sweets

Blackberries	8
Blackcurrants	8
Eating apples	10
Greengages	13
Gooseberries	5
Grapes, black	14
Grapes, green	17
Loganberries	5
Melons	4
Oranges	8
Pears	9
Plums	10
Prunes, raw	38
Raspberries	7
Rhubarb (fresh)	1
Stoned dates	70
Strawberries	7
Tinned fruit salad	20
Tinned pineapple	18
Tinned pears	18
Ice cream	56
Jam or marmalade	74
Jelly cubes	73

It will be seen from the above that the best sweet dishes a slimmer can eat are raw fruits. Any made-up sweet is very heavy on calories: a small apple pie, for example is 216 calories. For a treat you can make up ice cream dishes such as Peach Melba, Raspberry Ripple, Banana Split and Pear Helène: any of these would work out at between 155 and 180 calories. The important thing is to have these special treats on days when your calorie intake from other dishes is low enough to permit it being done without exceeding your overall total of 1,500 calories per day.

It is possible to save calories by making your own jellies out of gelatine flavoured with cordial and sweetened with saccharine. These would have a considerably lower calorie value than the shop product made from jelly cubes. Rice pudding etc can also be made with saccharine and the saving on sugar will dramatically cut the calories.

You may think $1\frac{1}{2}$oz of butter per day is a very meagre ration, but it is in fact rather more than the adult population existed upon during the last war. If you find $\frac{1}{2}$pt of milk simply does not go round for your tea, coffee and sweets, you can double the quantity if you use dried milk instead. One pint of dried milk made up has the same calorie value as $\frac{1}{2}$pt of fresh.

Vary your salads as suggested in Chapter 4, otherwise you will soon tire of them.

These menus do not allow for any alcoholic drinks in the day. If you are trying to slim, you must give up drinking, as the calorie value of most alcoholic drinks would make it impossible to reach your target of 1500 calories per day. As an example of what you would be up against, consider the following calorie values:

Alcoholic drinks		*Calorie values*
Brown ale		180 per pt
Draught bitter		180 ,,
Lager and lime		180 ,,
Sweet cider		240 ,,
Guinness		201 ,,
Whisky	standard pub measure	60 per single measure
Rum	standard pub measure	75 per single measure
Gin	standard pub measure	55 per single measure
Sherry, dry	standard pub measure	65 per $3\frac{1}{2}$fl oz
Sherry, sweet	standard pub measure	75 ,,
Port	standard pub measure	180 per wine glass (4 fl oz)
Sauternes		110 ,,
Beaujolais		80 ,,

Three pints of beer would be 540 calories which is equivalent in value to lunch or dinner. Which would you prefer? Even if you answer that you would prefer to miss the meal, you must not do that as it will result in your lacking essential nutrients.

You must get into the habit of seeing every dish in terms of its calorie value, and of doing the sums needed to balance your calorie account for the day. To help you do this, there is an excellent book published by HMSO at 55p for the use of caterers. It is called *Ready Reckoner of Food Values*. You will find in this far more information on particular foods than it is possible to include in a book of this size.

WHEN YOU REACH YOUR IDEAL WEIGHT

You cannot follow a strict diet for ever. When you have reduced to your ideal weight, you must make adjustments because if you continued on your reducing diet you would go on losing weight and so become underweight. You need to level out, as it were.

Do not, of course, go back at once to the things you were eating before. In a few weeks this would undo all your efforts. Instead, try allowing yourself little extras, perhaps a larger portion, and by experiment find out exactly how much you can allow yourself and still hold your weight steady. Weigh once a week; ignore day-to-day variations, even if you notice them. If your weight starts to increase, you are allowing yourself too much. If your weight decreases, you can take a little more. Only personal experiment will tell you what you can do to hold your weight steady, but with your experience of diet so far, you will have little difficulty in working out what is right for you.

The main things we cut out in the reducing diet were cereals, marmalade or other preserves at breakfast, and soups at dinner. Apart from that you were eating the same dishes as the rest of your family, following the menus in chapter 4. You could for a start, therefore, allow yourself soup again, or marmalade; you could have an extra slice of toast; or another ounce of fish or meat. It would be unwise to increase your bread or potato intake too much, however; it is preferable to increase other items.

TRIMMING THE MIDDLE-AGE BULGE

The exercise routines given in chapter 3 increase muscle tone and promote all-round fitness. For people who are troubled with fat in the wrong places, however, there are additional exercises that will help. It is mostly the middle aged who suffer with this problem. They develop a 'spare tyre' around their waist. In recent years, some of the young people have proved prone to this fatness as well, partly owing to lack of exercise and partly owing to overindulgence in alcohol.

The following exercises will help to correct this condition in people of all ages. They should be performed in addition to the exercises in chapter 3. I repeat, in addition.

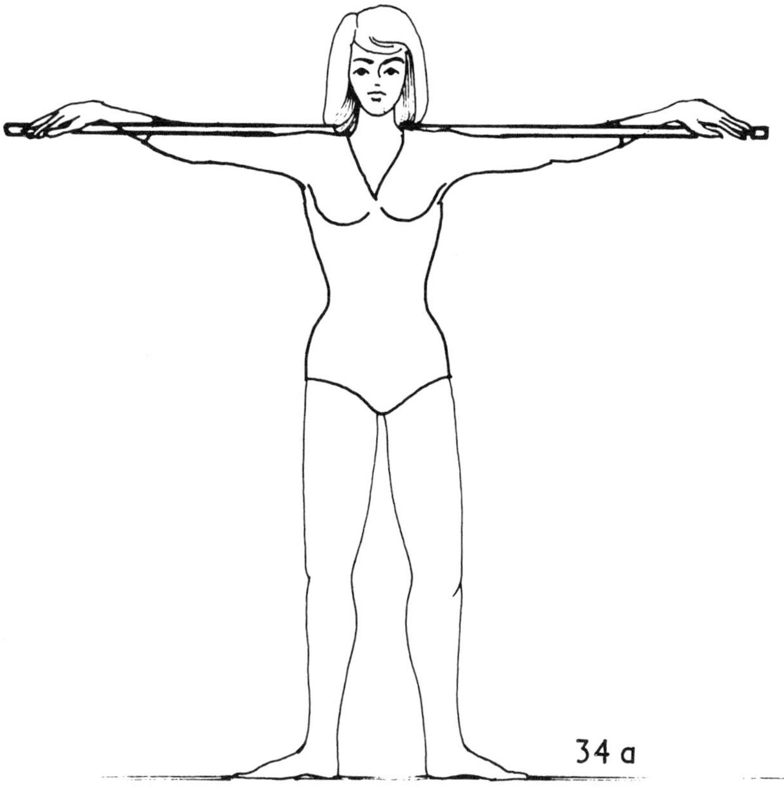

34 a

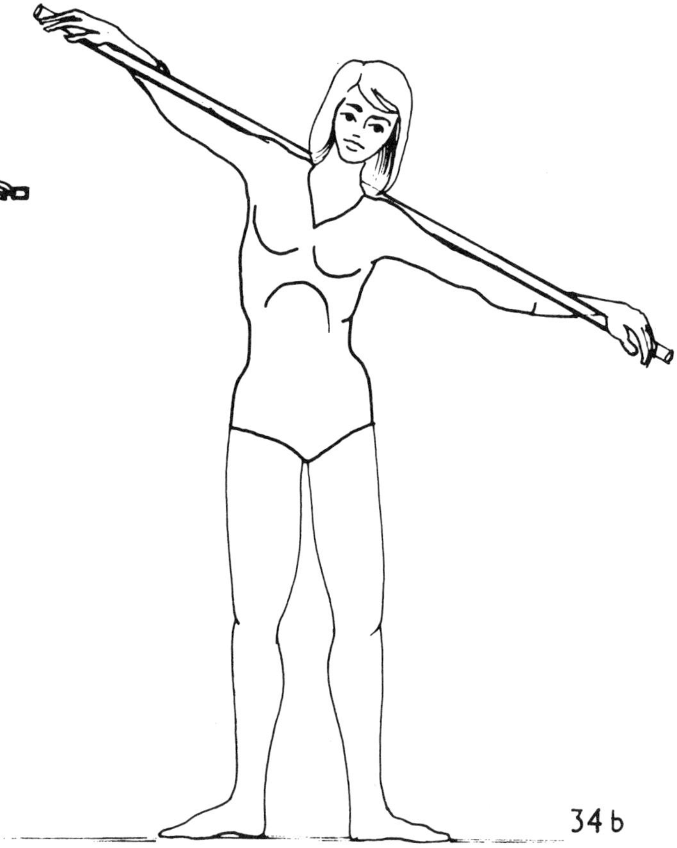

34 b

EXERCISE 1

Hold a broomstick across your shoulders behind your neck (Fig. 34a). Now bend over as far to your left side as possible (Fig. 34b). Straighten up and then bend over as far to your right side as possible. Straighten up.

Do ten repetitions each side.

EXERCISE 2

Take the broomstick across the back of your neck again as in exercise 1 (Fig. 34a). Turn as far to your left as possible (Fig. 34c). Come back to the front-facing position and then turn to your right as far as possible.

Do ten repetitions each side.

EXERCISE 3

Lie on your back. Raise your legs straight up in the air, supporting your hips on your hands and with your elbows on the ground (Fig. 35). Now perform a cycling action with your legs for 1 minute. Lower and rest. Then do another minute, lower and rest and then a third minute. As you progress and feel the ability, do longer periods.

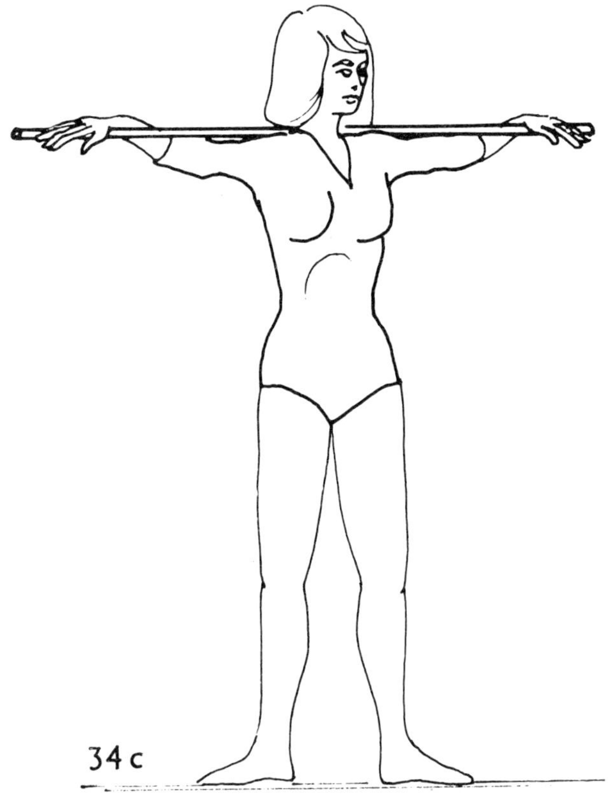

34c

35

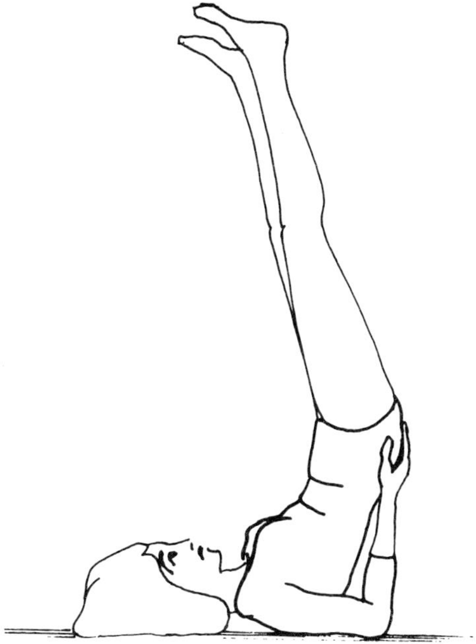

EXERCISE 4

Take up the position shown in Fig. 35. Slowly part your legs as far as possible sideways. Then bring them together again slowly. Perform the exercise with a slow, controlled movement.

Do ten repetitions.

36a

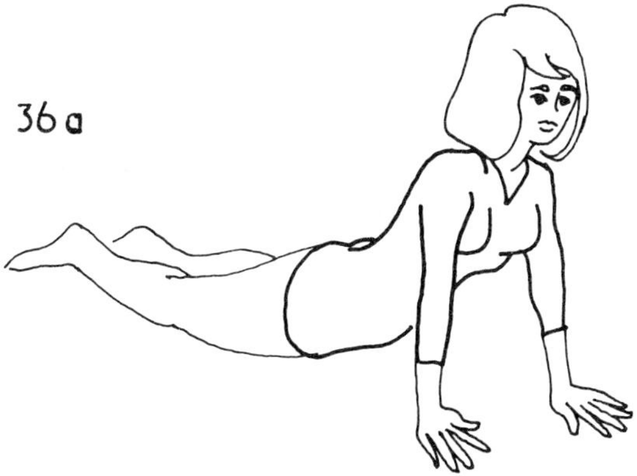

36b

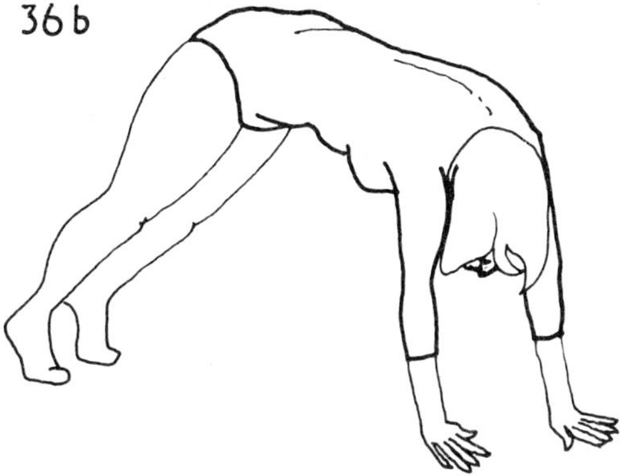

EXERCISE 5

Place the palms of your hands on the ground, fingers facing forwards, and have your toes on the ground. Lower your body, arching your back inwards in a hollow, with your chest upright (Fig. 36a). This posture is known as 'the cobra' in yoga. Now arch your back outwards, lowering your head, in the action known as the 'cat stretch' (Fig. 36b). Return to the first position.

Do ten repetitions.

EXERCISE 6

Stand feet astride, hands on hips (Fig. 37). Keep your hips square to the front and turn as far to your left as possible. Come back to the front-facing position and then turn as far to your right as possible.

Do ten repetitions each side.

EXERCISE 7

You need a bar or a beam for this one, as suggested in Chapter 3 (p. 46). Hang from the bar by the arms, with arms straight. Now raise your knees to your chest (Fig. 38) and then lower them to the straight position again.

Do ten repetitions.

EXERCISE 8

Hang with straight arms from the beam as in the last exercise. Now slowly raise both legs to the horizontal position straight out in front of you (Fig. 39). Lower and then raise again.

Do ten repetitions.

This is a more difficult exercise than the previous one. If you find it impossible initially, try the previous exercise for a month or so and then go on to this one.

EXERCISE 9

Lie on your back. Put your feet on a low stool, about 12–18in off the ground. Tie a strap or belt around the stool, with a loop into which you can tuck your feet. If need be put a weight on the stool to hold it down (Fig. 40a). Your arms should be above your head. Now swing your arms up to touch your toes, breathing out as you do so. (Fig. 40b). Lower to the floor, breathing in as you do so.

Do ten repetitions.

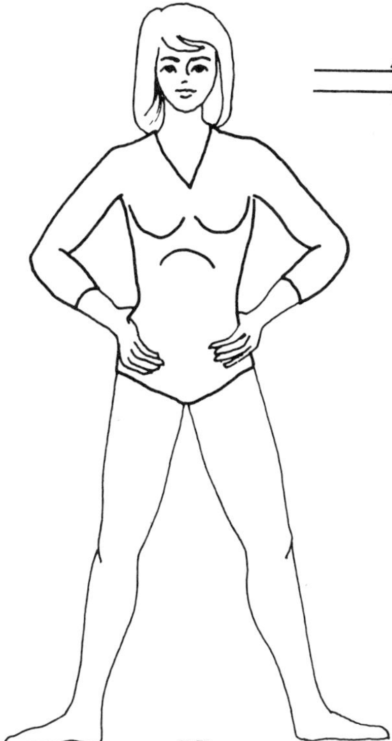

37

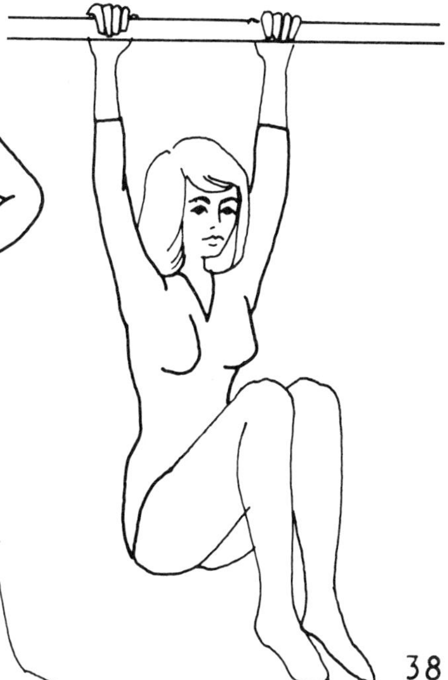

38

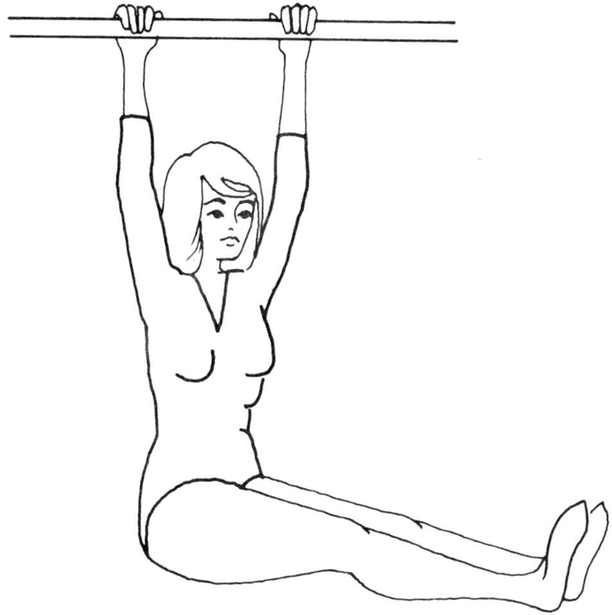

39

40a

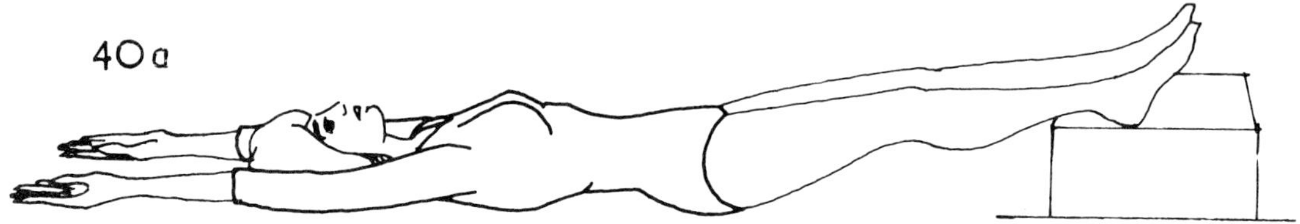

40b

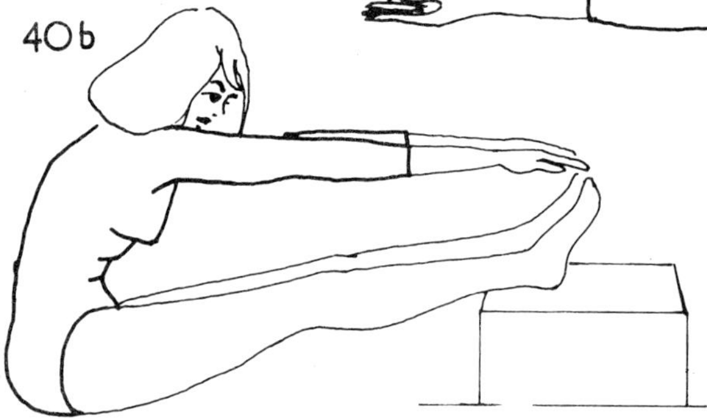

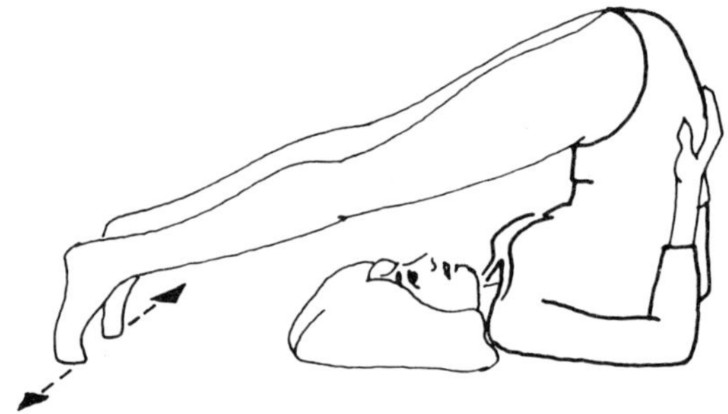

41

EXERCISE 10

Lie on your back. Raise your legs up in the air, supporting your hips with your hands and with your elbows on the ground (Fig. 35). Now take your feet right over to touch the floor (Fig. 41). The exercise from this position is to move the left foot one step to the left and then to close it back. Then the right foot one step to the right and close it back.

Do ten repetitions with each foot.

This again is an advanced exercise, and if you cannot do it at first, practice with number 3 for a month or two, and then try this one again.

EXERCISE 11

Skip for three minutes.

Taken with the full routine in Chapter 3, these eleven exercises should overcome the bulge problem.

6
The Problem of Underdevelopment

Underdevelopment used to concern the male more frequently than the female. Many young men resorted to advertised courses of training to build up their muscles. Today, with ladies participating in sport to a greater extent, they too can be conscious of a lack of muscular development, Being thin is usually regarded as a virtue in a woman but is often thought of as showing lack of strength in a man. Almost all young men who are underweight or undersized would like to improve, if they were honest about it.

There is no need for anyone to accept an underdeveloped physique. It is true that once you have passed the age of twenty-six you cannot alter your bone structure as you have finished growing, but the muscles can be developed, and doing so will make a surprising difference to your appearance, strength and general health.

The problem of developing muscles is rather different from the task of simply keeping fit. This is because of the way in which development takes place. You exercise vigorously in order to break down tissue, and nature, in replenishing that tissue, builds a little more than you have broken down. You must allow time for this reconstruction. When it has taken place, you exercise vigorously again in order to break down more tissue, and again nature rebuilds a little more, so that each time the particular muscle grows slightly. The two important points are that you must exercise to the limit of your capacity in order for this breakdown to occur, and you must rest as long as is needed for the rebuilding to take place. In order to develop your physique, therefore, you must not train every day, but every other day. This is most important.

You must also train regularly. It is of no use to put off exercising one night and tell yourself that you will do twice as much the next night to make up for it. Even if you carried out your promise, you would do more harm than good since you would overstrain yourself.

If you are aiming to build up your physique, you will need more food than normally. You must increase your protein intake, since protein builds muscle. Eat more meat, fish, eggs and dairy products and drink more milk. Your appetite will increase when you train, and will guide you as to the quantities of food you need. Continue to eat a balanced diet as recommended in Chapter 4, but increase your helpings of the protein foods.

The general rules as to how and when we should exercise given in Chapter 3 apply equally to the routines in this chapter with the one exception that now the exercises are only to be done every other day. Exercise in fresh air, with the window open if possible. Wear as little as possible and exercise in front of a mirror. Wait an hour and a half after a meal before beginning.

In most of the exercises in this chapter you will be told to do three sets. You must do the movement until you absolutely cannot do another. Then rest a minute and try again, going on until you cannot do another. Then rest a minute and do yet a third set until you cannot do another. As an example, you might find that in the first set you will manage ten movements, in the second set eight movements, and in the third set six movements. Each time you must work the muscle concerned to its absolute limit of endurance. You will find that with progress the number of repetitions rises, so that your ten, eight and six become eleven, nine and seven.

Weight-trainers exercise with weights on a dumb-bell rod or a bar, and when they reach the point where the number of repetitions they are doing is excessive, they simply put more weights on the dumb-bell and thus reduce the number of repetitions again. Similarly, people who train with chest expanders add another spring as their strength increases. If we are exercising without apparatus, we can overcome the excessive number of repetitions by moving on to a more difficult variation of the exercise.

The schedule given in this chapter can be followed by ladies as well as men, and if carried out regularly it will build up muscles. Do not expect results to become apparent immediately, however. The process is a long one and patience is needed.

It is encouraging to take your measurements before you begin training, and then again after three months, when you should begin to see results. After that, take your measurements at monthly intervals. You will certainly see improvements, small though they may be, and this will give you encouragement to go on; but turning an undersized body into a normal one may take two or three years, and it is important not to give up in despair too soon.

The measurements normally taken are as follows:

1 Across the chest, over the nipples. Breathe out and take the measurement with all the air expelled from your lungs. Then breathe in and take the measurement with the lungs full. The difference between the two measurements, ie the capacity of the lungs, is more important than the actual chest size.

2 The waist.

3 The biceps (upper arm). Take with the arm straight and then with the arm bent.

4 The lower arm.

5 The wrist.

6 The thigh.

7 The calf.

8 The neck.

9 The ankle.

10 Your height.

It is clearly easier if you can get someone to take the measurements for you, but if you cannot, do it in front of a mirror and try to read the tape in the mirror, so that you are not bending forwards to see the figures and so falsifying the readings.

All these measurements should show some slight improvement. Obviously the biggest changes will be in the chest and arm measurements, but the leg measurements will also improve. The wrist, ankle and height will show the least response, but the height may improve with better posture.

The following is the schedule of exercises to follow. As you will see it is largely based on the keep-fit routine of Chapter 3 and uses no apparatus except what would be found in the normal home.

EXERCISE 1 DEEP BREATHING

This is exactly the same as number 1 in Chapter 3, but this time, when you have done ten, breathe normally for about half a minute and then do another ten. Then breathe normally for half a minute and do a third set of ten.

This exercise, or the alternatives to it given in Chapter 3, can be followed throughout the course. There is no progression to a harder variation.

The importance of the exercise is that it will increase the lung capacity and will push out the walls of your chest, thus making it bigger from within. Coupled with the development of muscle from without, this can lead to a very gratifying increase in chest measurement, a point of great importance to the youth or man who is self-conscious about his slightness.

EXERCISE 2

This is the same as number 2 in Chapter 3, not the variation. When you have done ten repetitions, however, rest a minute and do ten more, and then rest a minute and do ten more.

EXERCISE 3

This is the same as number 3 in Chapter 3, or the given variation, whichever you prefer. Do ten repetitions each way, rest a minute and do ten more, and rest another minute and do ten more.

EXERCISE 4

This is the same as number 4 in Chapter 3, but this time it is done as a progressive exercise. The first time, you may find that you can lower and raise yourself ten times. Rest a minute and try again. This time you may manage eight. Rest a minute and try a third time. This time you may only do six. These figures are just an indication of what a normal man would do. If you can do more, you must, pushing yourself to your limit. If less, you must still go to your own personal limit. The essential thing is to push yourself until you just cannot continue, ie until you try and actually fail. It is the final one that you just cannot manage that does the good.

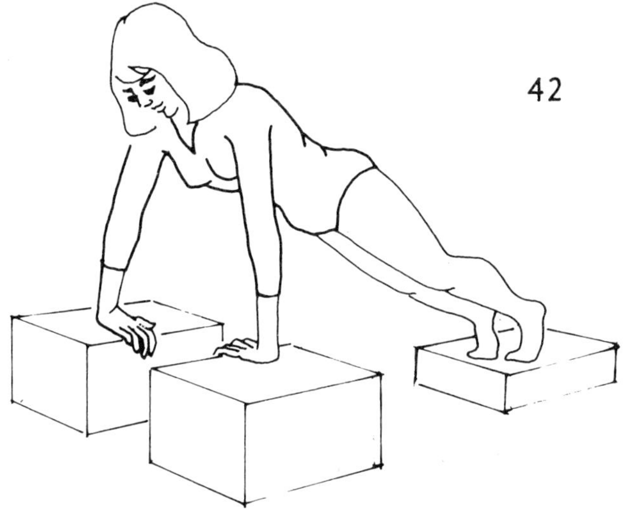

42

As you become stronger, you will find that the numbers you are doing rise. You may start at ten, eight and six, but soon you will be doing fifteen, twelve and ten.

You need a harder variation then to reduce your numbers. Try the exercise with the feet on a chair or stool and the hands on the seats of two others, placed shoulder width apart (Fig. 42). Lower yourself as far as possible.

A still harder variation to progress to is performing the movement with a weight on your back, such as a heavy book. Yet a further progression is to do four sets instead of three. All these progressions will enable you to make the exercise harder and harder, the stronger you become.

Do three sets to limit to begin with, and then increase to four sets to limit.

EXERCISE 5

This is the same as number 5 in Chapter 3, but again you must do three sets to limit. Lift the chair as many times as you possibly can, slowly; rest a minute, and do a second set, and rest another minute and do a third set. As a progression when you become stronger, use a heavier chair.

EXERCISE 6

To develop the biceps and triceps in this exercise and the next, it would be most convenient if you could make yourself some form of bar-bell. As this course is designed for the ordinary housewife or her husband, making use of things at hand, I would suggest that the simplest way to make what you want is to take a stout broomstick and to attach a weight to each end. A plastic bag of sand tied firmly to each end would do nicely.

Take your improvised bar-bell in both hands, hands shoulder width apart, palms facing away from your body (Fig. 43a). Now bring the bar to your shoulder level by bending your arms (Fig. 43b). This is the exercise that weight-trainers call 'curling'. Breathe out as you bend your arms, and in as you straighten them again to lower the bar-bell to arm's length.

Curl the bar again and lower again. Do as many repetitions as you possibly can, and then put the bar-bell down for a one minute rest. Try a second set, again doing as many as you possibly can before putting the bar down for another minute's rest. Then try a third set, again doing as many as you possibly can.

You should use a weight sufficiently heavy to make your number of possible repetitions work out at about ten, eight and six to begin with. If you find you are doing more, then you need a heavier weight. If you are only managing five or six on the first attempt, then you need a lighter weight initially.

When the number of repetitions you can do on your first set rises above fifteen, change the weight to a slightly heavier one. It is usual to add 5lb to the weight each time you increase it.

EXERCISE 7

Hold your improvised bar-bell behind you, arms shoulder width apart and palms facing front (Fig 44a). Now, without leaning forwards, try to raise the bar backwards keeping the arms straight. You will find that you will only be able to move it a few inches from your body (Fig. 44b). Breathe out as you raise the bar, and in as you lower. Do as many as you possibly can, rest a minute, do as many as you possibly can again, rest a minute, and then do as many as you can a third time.

As a progression, add to the weight as your strength increases.

EXERCISE 8

Make a wrist roller as follows. Take a short piece of round wood, such as a sawn off piece of a broomstick, about 12in long. Tie a piece of stout cord around the

43a

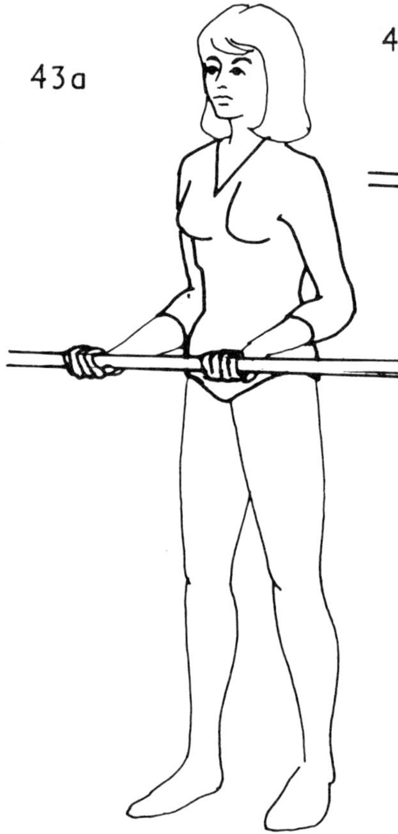

43b

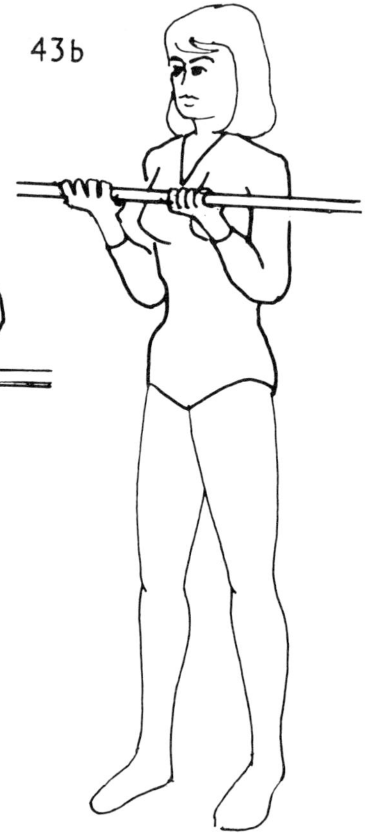

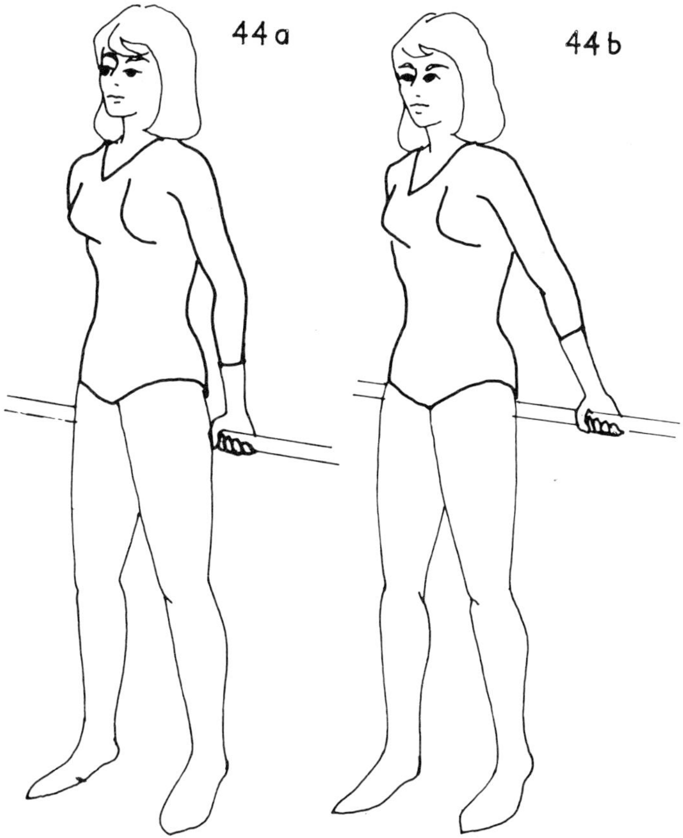

middle and fasten it to the stick with a nail or screw so that it will not slip around. The cord should be about 3ft long. Hang a weight to the end of the cord.

The exercise is to hold the rod out at arm's length in front of you, shoulder height, one hand grasping each end of the wood (Fig. 45). The weight hangs down and you have to raise it up by turning the roller with your hands, so winding the cord around it. Wind it up and lower and wind again as many times as you can, but do one set only, not three as in the former exercises.

As a progression, use a heavier weight.

EXERCISE 9

This is exactly the same exercise as number 9 in Chapter 3, but you perform it holding a weight in each hand. A stone, a half brick or even a heavy book would do (Figs. 11a, 11b and 11c). Do twenty each side, rest a minute, then another twenty, rest a minute, and then a third twenty.

Add a repetition each week until you are doing forty in each set.

EXERCISE 10

This is exactly the same as number 10 in Chapter 3, but do three sets of twenty each side with a minute's rest between each set (Figs. 12a, 12b and 12c). Add one repetition each side per week until you are doing forty each side.

EXERCISE 11

This is exactly the same as number 11 in Chapter 3 (Figs. 13a and 13b). Do as many repetitions as you can manage. You will find it begins to hurt the abdominal region, but force yourself to go on to the limit. Rest a minute and try a second set to the limit, and then rest again and try a third set to the limit. Remember that it is the one you just cannot manage that is doing you good. You will probably manage something like twenty, fifteen and ten in the three sets at the beginning. Continue until you are doubling those numbers.

Then, as a progression, try the same exercise but instead of starting with the arms above the head as in Fig. 13a, hold a heavy book or other suitable weight at the back of your head. You will see that this adds to the weight you are raising and so exercises the

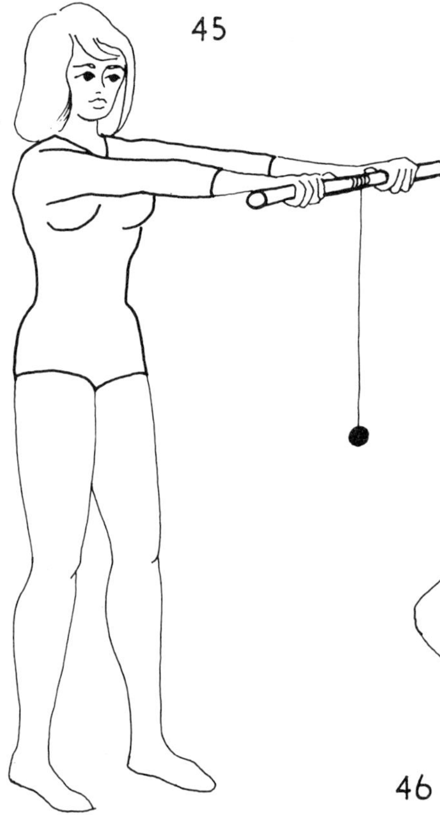

45

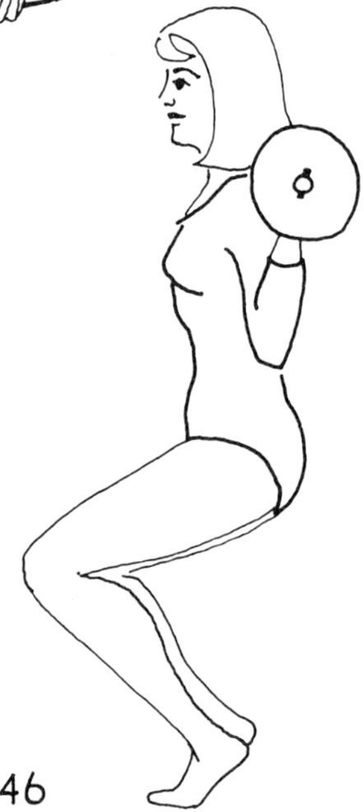

46

abdominal muscles even more strongly. You can continue making the exercise harder all the time by increasing this weight.

EXERCISE 12

This is exactly like number 12 in Chapter 3 for the lower abdominals (Figs. 14a, 14b and 14c). Do as many repetitions as you possibly can, rest a minute, do a second set, rest a minute, and then do a third set. You can lower your heels to the floor for your one minute's rest, but keep them off the floor during your set.

As a progression, try the exercise with heavy shoes or boots on your feet, thus increasing the work on your muscles. Weight-trainers actually use iron boots with weights attached to them.

As a further progression to this most important exercise, do both the variations described in Chapter 3 (Figs. 31 and 32). In each case do three sets to limit.

EXERCISE 13

This is exactly the same as the variation to number 13 in Chapter 3 (Figs. 33a and 33b).

Do ten repetitions only, since it is an exercise for suppleness rather than for development.

EXERCISE 14

This is the same as number 14 in Chapter 3 (Figs. 16a and 16b). Do as many as you can manage, rest a minute, do a second set, rest a minute, and then try a third set. Once you find them too easy, progress to performing the exercise with a weight in each hand, eg a half brick. As a further progression, try the exercise while holding a heavier weight, such as a sandbag, across the back of your neck (Fig. 46).

Because it encourages you to take deep breaths, this exercise is quite good for developing the chest as well as the leg muscles which it is primarily designed to exercise.

EXERCISE 15

This is exactly the same as number 15 in Chapter 3 (Fig. 17). Do ten repetitions only as it is for suppleness rather than added strength, and the ankles are also getting quite a lot of benefit from the last exercise.

EXERCISE 16

Repeat number 1 of this routine – the deep breathing. This relaxes you and is of vast benefit in itself.

This completes your course. You will need patience to follow it for a year or two to see really spectacular development in your physique, as worthwhile improvements are not built in a day or a month. But have faith and perserverance, and development cannot fail to take place.

7
Exercises for Odd Moments

Some people may feel that tying themselves to a routine of exercise every day will be too fatiguing. Once the habit became established they would find in fact that this was not so. The general benefits and the increased fitness would make their work-out a pleasure instead of a chore. However, there are exercises which can be done at any odd moment in the day, and if care were taken to exercise all the muscles and not only just a few, then these exercises could replace the routine given in Chapter 3. More usefully, of course, they could be used to supplement the routine in Chapter 3.

The housewife at her sink, the typist at her desk, the businessman caught in a traffic jam and sitting idly at the wheel of his car, could all use their wasted moments with beneficial exercise, and whether these odd exercises added up during the day to a full routine or were simply supplementary to the main evening routine, they would help in promoting fitness.

Many people experience special problems about exercising. Travellers cannot carry any apparatus and with only an hotel room at their disposal they have very little space. Single people living in lodgings find that anything vigorous or noisy might bring objections from their landlady or other lodgers. For people in these situations the routines given in this chapter might prove to be suitable alternatives to those in Chapter 3.

The system of exercising which can help in all these cases is known as 'isometrics'. Isometrics is a system of training which does not involve making large movements of the muscles or limbs. You simply try to make movements but prevent yourself from doing so by applying your effort to an immovable object or to contrary effort of another muscle. The simplest example of an isometric exercise is pushing against a wall. You will not push the wall over but you will develop your arm muscles by trying.

Isometrics started in America but the method is rapidly becoming established in Europe now. Amongst others who have used this method are the US Marines and Olympic athletes.

As I have stressed earlier in this book, it is

absolutely essential to get all-round exercise. Do not concentrate on building big arms or a big chest and neglect some other part of your body. Do not do just those exercises that you like, as these will be those you find easiest and the mere fact that you do find them easy shows that they are the ones you least need.

In this chapter, therefore, we shall first give a complete all-round routine for every muscle. This will suit someone who can only train by isometric methods for one of the reasons suggested above. We shall then consider supplementary exercises that could be used as additions to the general routine in Chapter 3.

GENERAL ISOMETRIC ROUTINE

The general rules for exercising given in Chapter 3 will apply as far as possible. If you are exercising at home wear as little as possible and see that you are getting plenty of fresh air during your training session. If you are in your car or at the office then, of course, you will have to exercise in whatever you happen to be wearing at the time, but still try to get fresh air.

The basic idea of isometrics is that you hold the contraction of a muscle (that is the effort you are making) for a count of six seconds. There is no advantage in holding it for more. The results do not improve proportionally. Neither is there any advantage in repeating the exercise. Experiments have shown that once a day for each exercise produces the effect desired, and that students who have done as many as seven repetitions have not had any better results. You must perform each exercise as hard or as strongly as you can without straining. In effect, doing this means that you are using 50 per cent of your full strength and this is correct. You must also exercise every day. It has been found that to miss a day and to train every other day reduces progress by as much as 20 per cent.

Since there are only sixteen exercises in the full routine you will see that the whole programme can be done in one and three-quarter minutes. Even allowing for the brief rests between exercises you would not take more than five minutes a day. This is clearly the system for the man or woman who hasn't got much energy or enthusiasm for ordinary methods.

Before you perform each isometric exercise, you take a deep breath and hold it for the duration of the six-second contraction. You then breathe out and rest a few seconds before the next exercise.

Since the isometric exercises do not include breath-

47

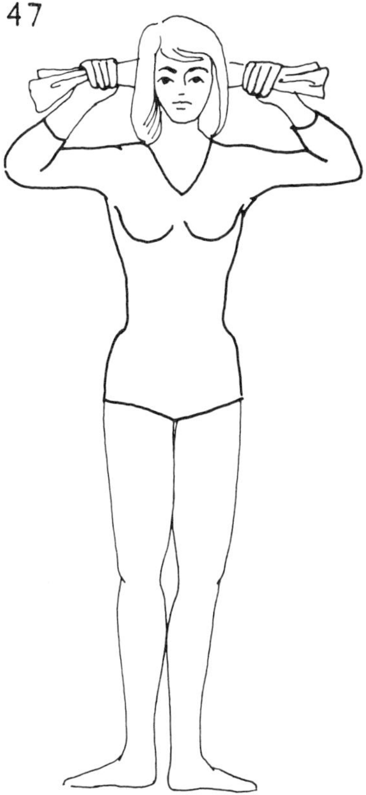

48

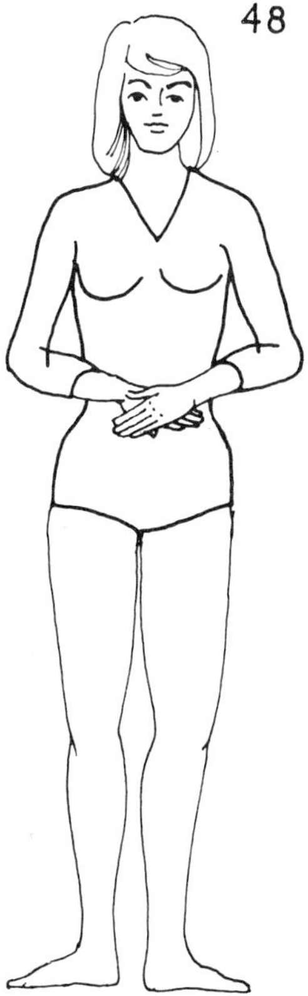

ing we must add to the routine numbers 1 and 16 from Chapter 3 to give completeness. The fourteen in between are purely isometric.

EXERCISE 1

This is deep breathing as in number 1 of Chapter 3 (Figs. 3a, 3b and 3c).

EXERCISE 2 FOR THE NECK MUSCLES

Take the ends of a towel, one in each hand, and put it behind your head. Have your elbows out in line with your shoulders (Fig. 47). With your hands pull the towel forwards, and with your head press back. Neither the hands nor the head actually move, since the effort of the hands is counteracted by the resistance of the head. Hold the effort for six seconds.

EXERCISE 3 FOR THE BICEPS AND TRICEPS

Stand upright. Bend the right arm at the elbow, holding the palm of the hand uppermost. Bring the left hand across the front of your chest and place it, palm downwards, on your right (Fig. 48). Now you press upwards with your right hand trying to raise the forearm by bending the elbow, and at the same time you prevent the movement being made by pressing down with your left hand. Neither arm must move. The pressure of one must counteract the effort of the other. The biceps will be exercised in your right arm and the triceps in your left.

Hold the effort for six seconds.

Repeat the movement with the opposite hands, ie the left pressing upwards and the right pressing downwards.

EXERCISE 4 FOR THE BICEPS AND TRICEPS

This is the opposite of the previous exercise and so varies the work for the muscles concerned. This exercise is beneficial and should not be omitted as being too similar to number 3.

Stand upright. Hold the left hand palm upwards across the front of your body and place the right fist in it (Fig. 49). Now try to press down with your right fist and prevent the movement by pressing up with your left hand. The effort of the one is frustrated by the resistance of the other and there is no actual movement. Hold the effort for six seconds.

Repeat the exercise with opposite hand.

49

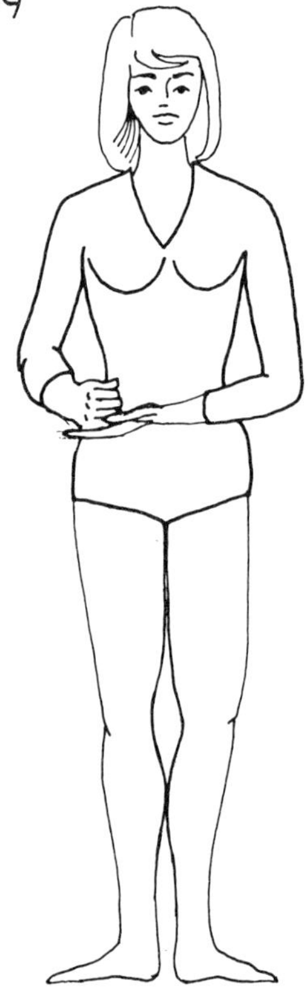

50

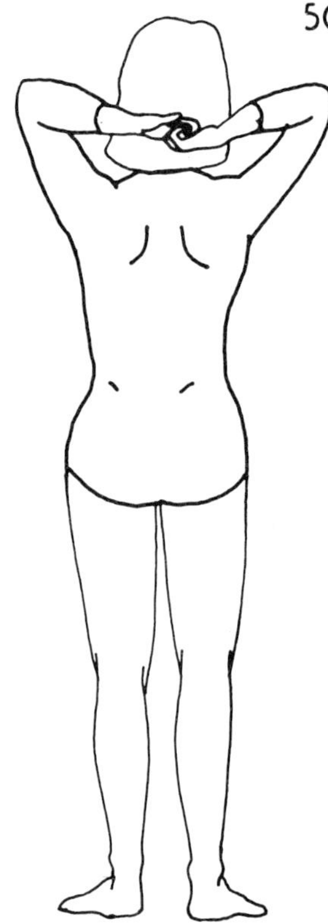

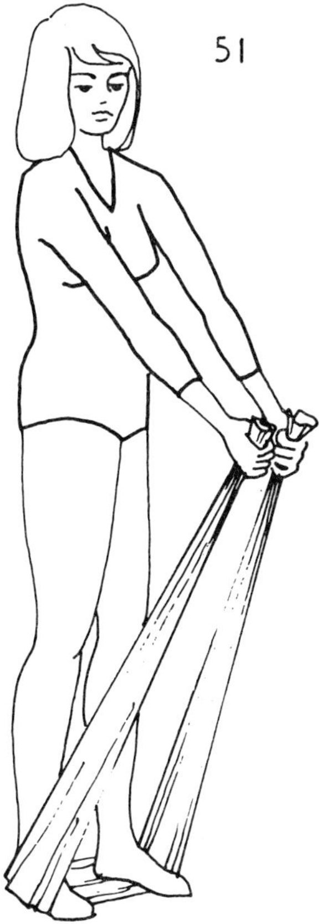

51

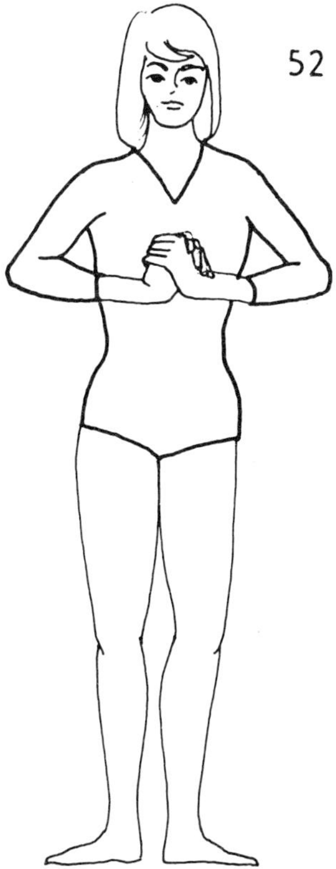

52

EXERCISE 5 FOR THE SHOULDERS

Clasp the hands behind your head by interlocking your fingers (Fig. 50). Try to pull the hands apart. The interlocked fingers prevent this, of course, but hold the effort as strongly as you can for six seconds.

EXERCISE 6 FOR THE DELTOIDS

Take a piece of rope, a canvas belt or a long towel. Place it under your feet so that you are standing on it. Hold one end in each hand (Fig. 51). Now try to raise your arms forwards and upwards, keeping them straight, as though you were going to raise them straight out in front of you at shoulder level. Do not lean forwards, but stay upright while making the effort. You will not be able to raise your arms since you will be pulling on the ends of the towel which is anchored under your feet. Hold the effort for six seconds.

EXERCISE 7 FOR THE PECTORALS

Raise your elbows to a horizontal position in front of you and clasp your hands in front of your chest by placing them palm to palm and bending the fingers over (Fig. 52). Now press your hands strongly together and hold the effort for a count of six. No movement will be made since the pressure of one hand is countered by the pressure of the other.

EXERCISE 8 FOR THE ABDOMINALS

Stand upright and take a deep breath. Now breathe out, emptying the lungs as much as possible, and at the same time pull the stomach in and up as far as it will go. Hold the effort and position for a count of six seconds (Fig. 53). This is the best known exercise for the 'middle-aged bulge' and it has the advantage that it can be done anywhere in a standing or sitting position. Do it once a day.

EXERCISE 9 FOR THE ABDOMINALS

Lie on your back. Raise the knees and bring the feet up so that the heels are as close to the buttocks as you can get them. Clasp your hands behind your head (Fig. 54). Now, from this position, try to sit up slowly. You will not be able to do so, but hold the effort for six seconds and you will find it is of great benefit.

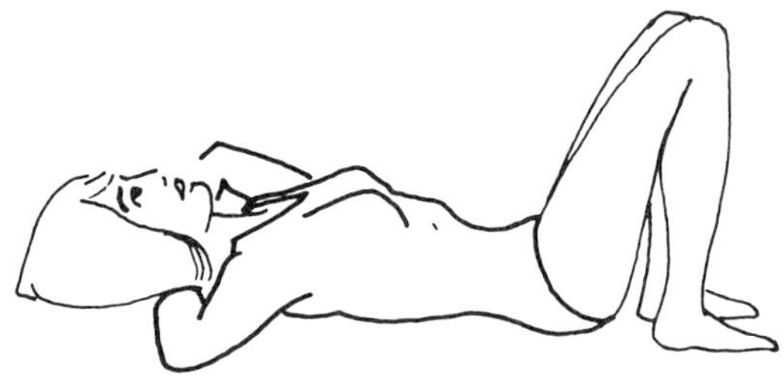

54

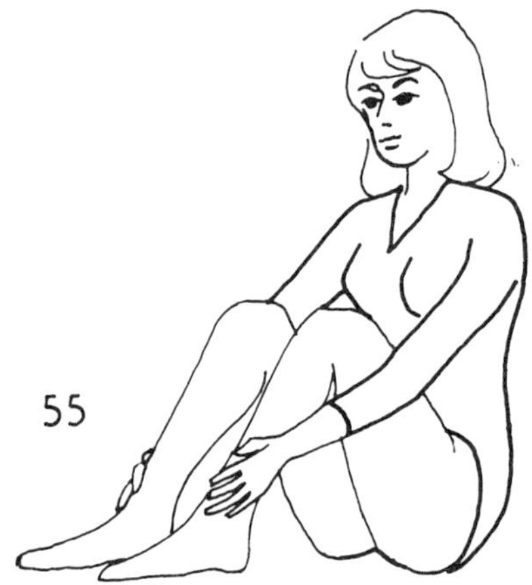

55

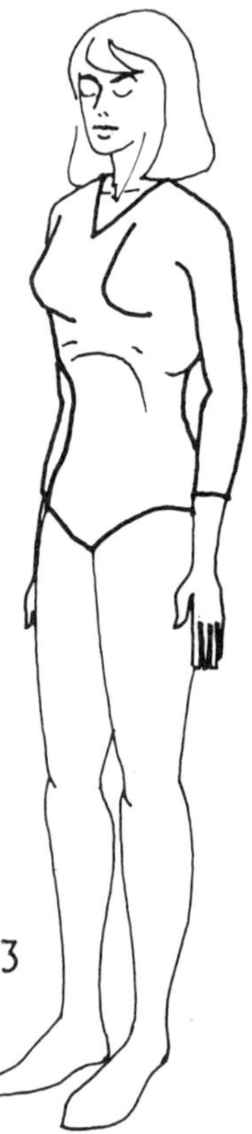

53

EXERCISE 10 FOR THE BACK

Sit upright on the floor with your feet on the ground and your knees up. Lean forwards and grasp your ankles with your hands (Fig. 55). Now pull back with your hands and resist by pushing forwards with your legs. Since your legs will probably be stronger than your arms, you will have to pull harder with your hands than you push. Do not move at all. Make the pull of the arms exactly balance the push of the legs. Hold the effort for six seconds.

EXERCISE 11 FOR THE HIPS

Sit on a chair. Grasp the seat on either side with your hands. Raise the legs off the ground and, keeping them straight out in front of you, cross the ankles. Lock one foot behind the other (Fig. 56). Now try to force the legs apart. You will not be able to do so, since the ankles are locked, but hold the effort for six seconds. If you are doing the exercise correctly you will feel the effort all up your legs, both in the calf muscles and in the thigh, and it will benefit the hip joint area as well.

Reverse your feet and repeat the exercise.

EXERCISE 12 FOR THE WHOLE BODY

Lie face down on the floor. Raise the feet and bend the body backwards so that you can grasp your ankles. This is exactly the same as the variation on number 13 in Chapter 3 (Fig. 33b). It is a yoga posture known as 'the bow'. Now bend your head back and bring your feet forwards, trying to make the back of your head meet the soles of your feet. You will not come anywhere near doing so, but hold the effort for six seconds.

EXERCISE 13 FOR THE LEG MUSCLES

Lie on your back. Raise your right leg so that the upper part is perpendicular and the lower part is parallel to the floor, the knee joint making a right angle. Loop a towel around your right foot, and hold one end in each hand (Fig. 57). Now try to straighten your right leg and resist the effort by pulling on the ends of the towel. No actual movement is possible, since the push of the foot is stopped by the pull on the towel, but hold the effort for six seconds.

Repeat with the left leg.

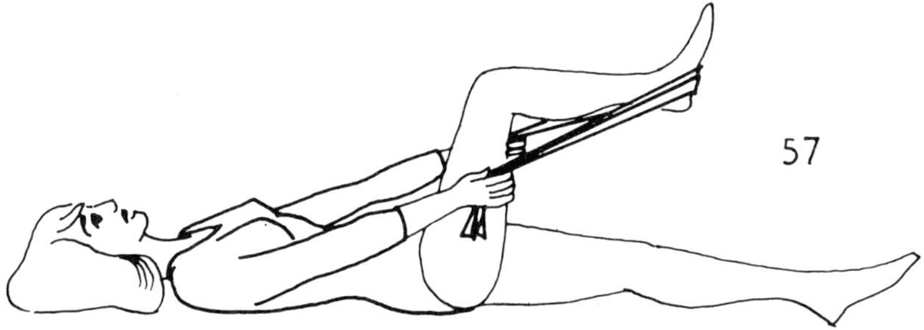

57

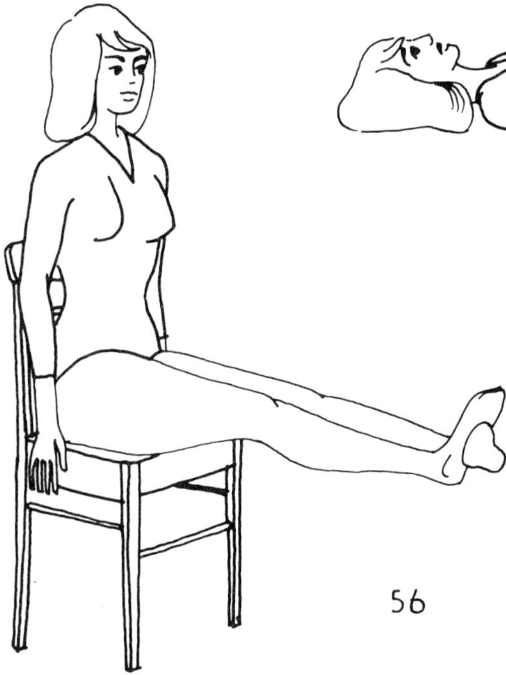

56

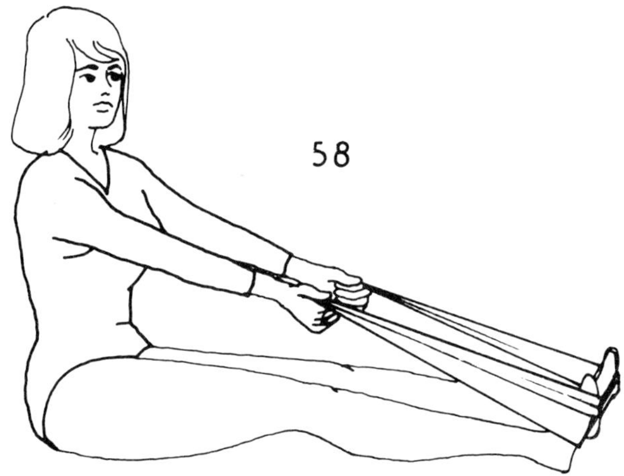

58

EXERCISE 14 FOR THE CALF MUSCLES

Sit upright on the floor with both legs stretched out straight in front of you. Loop a towel around your toes, feet together, and take one end in each hand (Fig. 58). Now try to point the toes and resist the attempt by pulling on the ends of the towel. Hold the effort for six seconds.

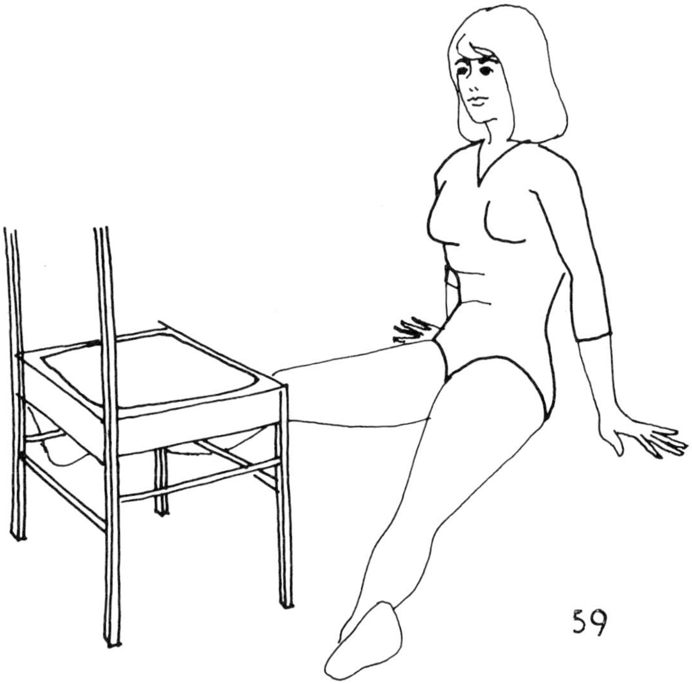

59

EXERCISE 15 FOR THE INNER THIGH MUSCLES

Sit upright on the floor with a chair between your feet. Raise your heels slightly off the ground, putting your hands on the ground behind you to give you balance (Fig. 59). Now squeeze in on the legs of the chair by trying to bring your legs together. Hold the effort for six seconds.

EXERCISE 16 BREATHING EXERCISE

Repeat exercise 1 of this schedule. Do not omit it, as finishing your routine with deep breathing helps you to relax, besides conferring benefit in itself.

The above routine gives an all-round work-out. We shall now consider exercises for odd moments which will be beneficial as supplementary exercises to Chapter 3 but which do not constitute a full routine in themselves.

ISOMETRICS IN THE KITCHEN

FOR ARMS AND SHOULDERS

Chair lift

Sit upright in a chair. Grasp the seat on either side with your fingers underneath. If you are not high enough to do this with straight arms, put a cushion or two in the chair (Fig. 60). Now breathe in deeply and hold your breath while you try to lift the seat upwards with your hands. Hold the effort for six seconds.

Curl under table

Sit by a heavy table. (If you have not got one heavy enough put some weight on it.) Place your hands under the edge of the table, palms upwards (Fig. 61). Breathe in and hold your breath while you try to lift the table with your hands, trying to bend the elbows to so. Do not make any actual movement at all: the table must be heavy enough to frustrate your effort. Hold the effort for six seconds.

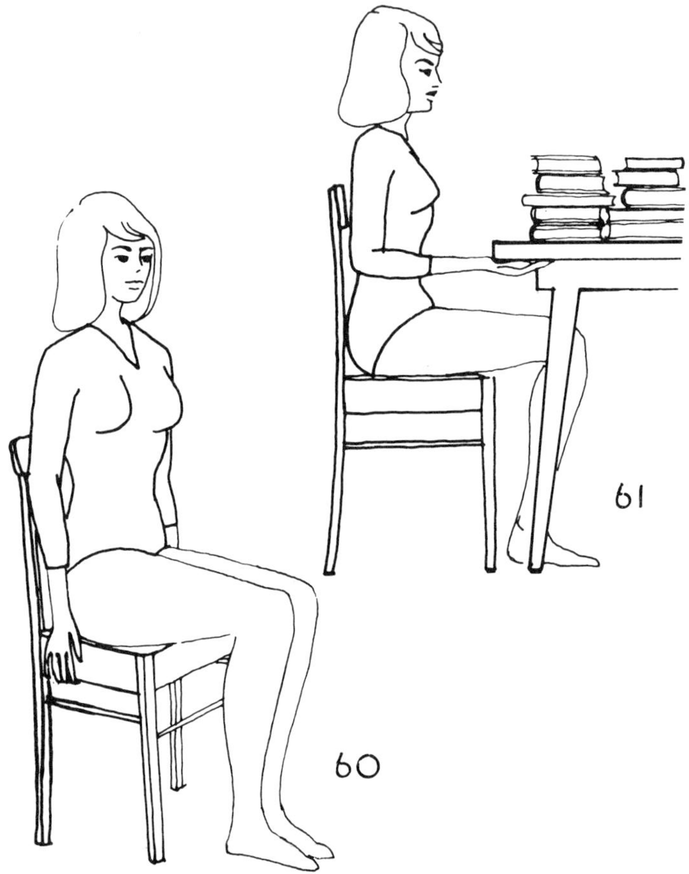

61

60

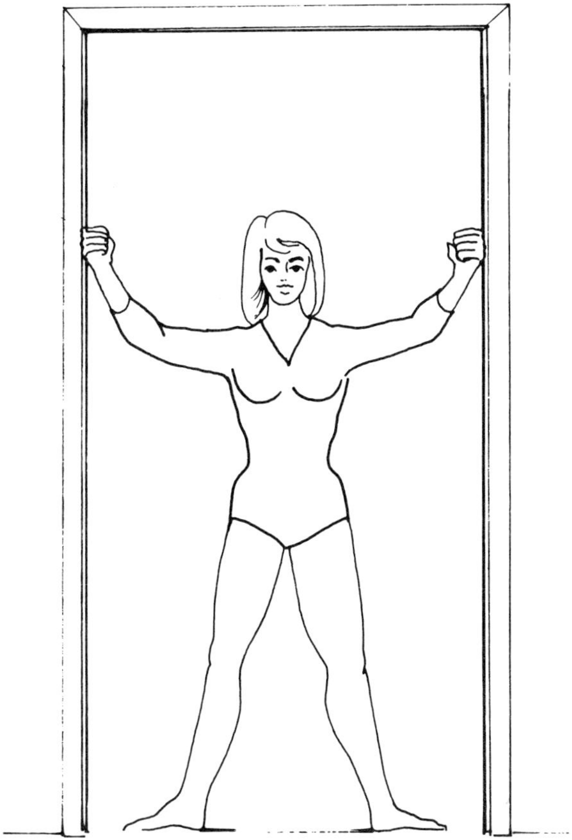

62

Press down on table

Sit at a table as before. This time place your hands flat on the top, palms downwards and just over the edge. Take a deep breath and while you hold your breath press down on the table top. Hold the effort for six seconds.

Outwards press in doorway

Stand in a doorway. Clench your fists and place the outside edges of your fists against the sides of the doorway (Fig. 62). Take a deep breath and press outwards with both fists for six seconds.

Upwards press in doorway

This is like the overhead press that weight-trainers do, and develops the same muscles.

Stand in a doorway and place the hands with palms upwards against the top of the frame, having your knees slightly bent while you do so. If you are tall enough you may be able to do this standing on the ground. If you are too short, stand on a stool or chair (Fig. 63). Breathe in, and whilst holding the breath, press upwards with both hands for six seconds. No movement is possible. It is the effort that counts.

Pull-over with chair

Lie on your back. Reach behind your head with both hands, arms straight, and grasp the legs of a heavy chair. Put weights on the chair or have someone sit on it if necessary to stop you lifting it (Fig. 64). Take a deep breath and whilst holding your breath try to lift the chair. Hold the effort for six seconds. Again there is no movement, only the effort.

Squeeze-in

This exercise can be done with practically any object that is firm enough. A door, a saucepan, an electric cooker, a wooden box are all suitable items. With arms straight out in front of you place one hand on each side of the chosen object, take a deep breath, and whilst holding your breath try to squeeze the object with the hands. Hold the effort for six seconds.

The crucifix with chairs

Lie on your back with arms straight out from the shoulders sideways. Place two heavy chairs so that you can grasp the bottom of the leg of each with one hand (Fig. 65). If the chairs are not heavy enough put weights on them or have someone sit on them. The

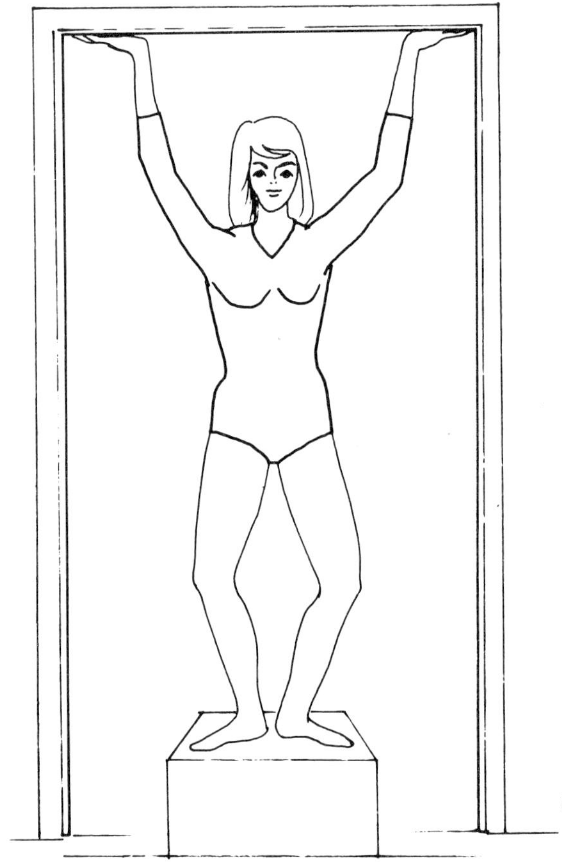

63

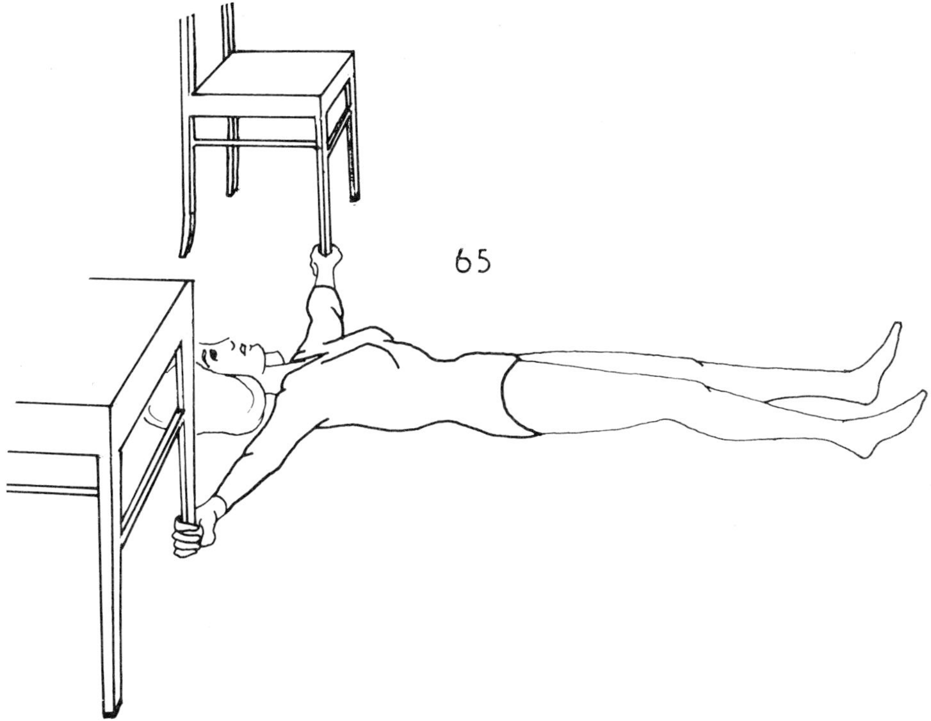

65

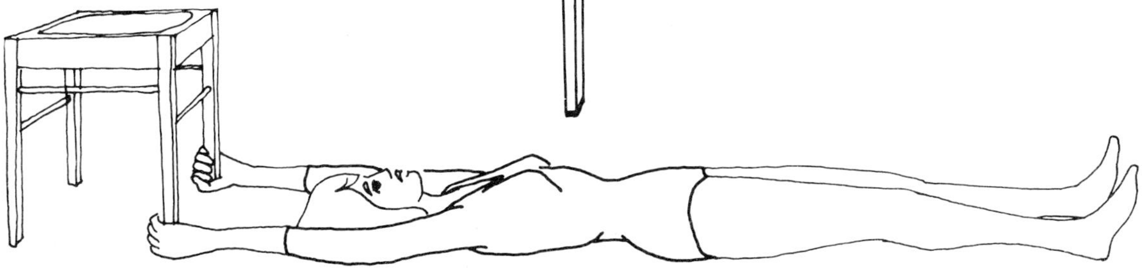

64

chairs must be heavy enough to stop you making any movement. Take a deep breath and while holding your breath, try to lift the chairs. Maintain the effort for a count of six seconds.

Press down

Turn a sweeping brush upside down and put the handle end on the floor with the handle upright. Place your hands on the top (Fig. 66). Take a deep breath and press down as hard as you can for six seconds.

FOR THE ABDOMINALS

The exercises listed in the last schedule, ie numbers 8 and 9 in this chapter, will be useful. Also the following:

The curl up

Lie on your back close to a wall. Raise your legs and place them against the wall, moving in closer if need be to enable you to do this. Clasp your hands behind your head (Fig. 67). Take a deep breath, and as you breathe out try to curl up by pulling your head off the ground with your clasped hands and raising your shoulders. Again it is an action you cannot perform, but hold the effort for six seconds.

FOR THE LEGS

Leg raises

Sit upright on the floor, with your hands on the ground behind you to support yourself. Stretch out your legs and put your left foot under the seat of a heavy chair, weighted down if necessary with a pile of books (Fig. 68). Take a deep breath, and while holding the breath try to raise the leg against the resistance of the seat of the chair. You will not be able to do so, but hold the effort for six seconds.

Repeat the exercise with the other leg.

Side foot raises

Stand about a foot away from a wall with your right side facing the wall. Place the outside of your right foot against the wall, keeping the leg straight (Fig. 69). Take a deep breath and hold the breath as you try to push sideways against the wall with the edge of your foot. You are in fact trying to raise your leg sideways but being prevented by the wall. Hold the effort for six seconds.

Repeat with your left side to the wall and your left leg pushing against the wall.

66

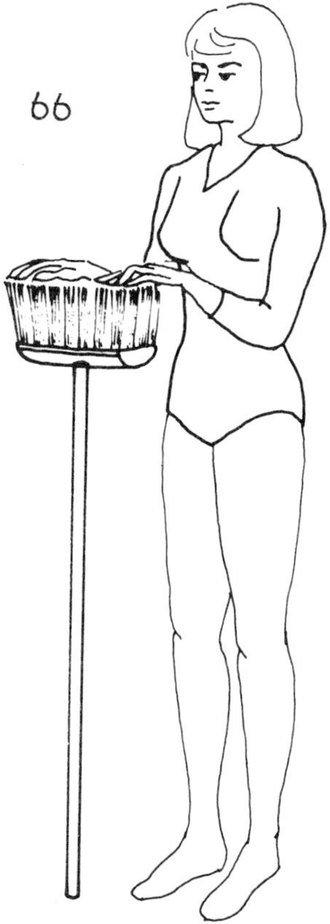

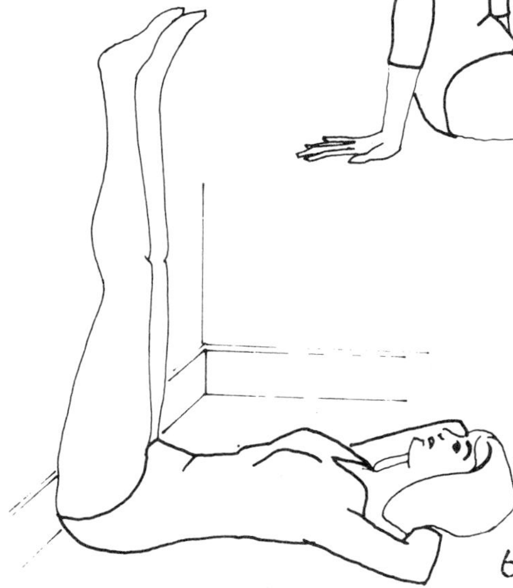

67

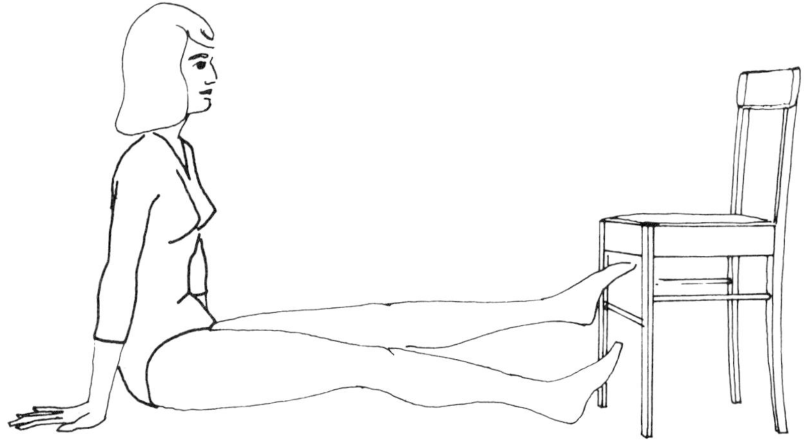

68

Back foot raises

Stand about a foot away from a wall with your back to the wall. Raise your right heel, and whilst remaining upright place the heel against the wall, keeping the leg straight. Take a deep breath and try to raise the right leg further backwards, pressing against the wall. Hold your breath and maintain the effort for six seconds.

Repeat the exercise with the left leg.

ISOMETRICS IN THE OFFICE

Most of the exercises given for the kitchen can be adapted for use in the office.

The chair lift will be possible, since you will have a chair in your office. The curl under table can be done at your desk as can the press down on table. The outwards and upwards press in doorway are possible and the squeeze-in can be done with your typewriter or a filing cabinet.

Obviously you will not want to do any of the lying down exercises in the office, but for the abdominals you can do number 8 of the all-round routine in this chapter (Fig. 53) seated at your desk. The side and

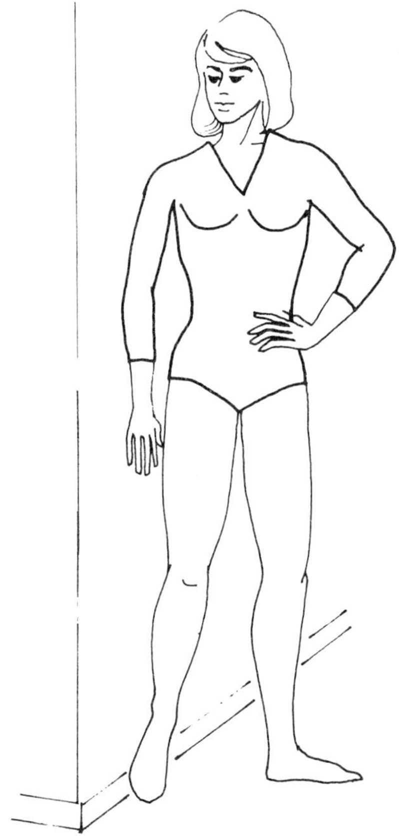

69

back foot raises also present no difficulty.

Additionally, seated at your desk, you can try the following:

Knee raises

Sitting at your desk, raise your right knee against the underside of your desk. Take a deep breath, and whilst holding the breath press upwards for six seconds. Repeat with the left knee.

Brow clasping

Rest your elbows on your desk. Place your palms one over the other against your forehead (Fig. 70). Take a deep breath and whilst holding the breath press forwards with your head and backwards with your hands, so that the effort of one neutralises the effort of the other. Hold the effort for six seconds.

70

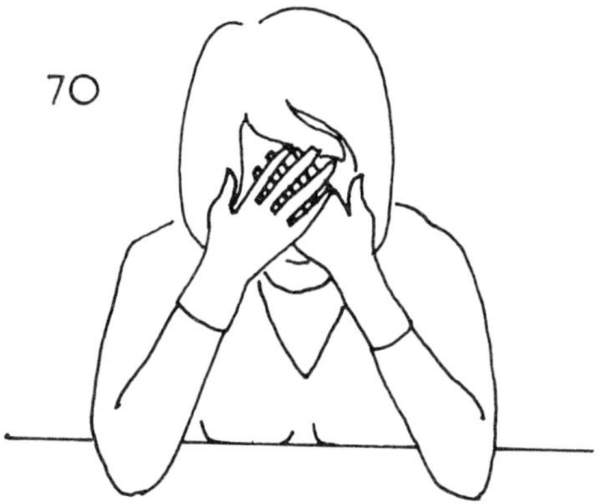

Head bending

Sit sideways at your desk with your right side to the desk. Place your right elbow on the top and your right hand on the right side of your head just over the ear. Take a deep breath, and whilst holding the breath press sideways with your head and hold your head up with your hand. The one effort neutralises the other and there is no movement, but hold the effort for six seconds.

Repeat with the left side against the desk and the left hand on the left side of the head.

ISOMETRICS IN THE CAR

Many of the above exercises can be adapted for use in your car in odd moments when you might be stationary in traffic or waiting for someone in a layby.

Exercise 8 in the all-round routine of this chapter

is clearly possible anywhere. The squeeze-in can be done on the steering wheel. The legs can be exercised by trying to straighten them against the floor. Remember to take a deep breath and to hold the breath and the effort for six seconds only. The curl under table can be performed with the hands under the dashboard, and the upwards press can be performed pushing against the roof of the car.

Once you become interested in isometrics you will be able to invent dozens of variations for yourselves, so that it can be said of these exercises that you can adapt them to wherever you happen to be and can use whatever implements you have to hand.

Any action of pushing or squeezing that is frustrated by the immovability of the object pushed or squeezed is essentially an isometric exercise. Any exercise that opposes one movement of your body against another so that stalemate results is an isometric exercise.

Remember three things:

1 Take a deep breath.
2 Hold the breath while making the effort.
3 Maintain the effort for six seconds only.

Do not expect to obtain double the benefit by doing more than is stated. Ten seconds effort is too long and produces fatigue. Four seconds is too short and does not produce satisfactory results. Six seconds has been found by trial to be the best. Do the exercises once a day and once only. Benefit will not increase in proportion to the number of repetitions. In fact it will not increase at all.

8
Additional Aids to Fitness

Some people find they have special problems over their diet. They may live in lodgings and have to eat what they are given with very little choice. Even men who live at home may have to take some meals in works canteens where the choice may be limited, though many canteens are improving to the extent of offering salad and even vegetarian dishes these days.

Anyone who does have these special difficulties will have to watch his or her health carefully. If you are becoming overweight, some form of dieting combined with exercise is essential. The less you can adjust your diet, the more you must adjust your exercise.

Probably the simplest adjustment of diet that is possible in most of these cases is to replace sandwiches or the canteen lunch in the middle of the day with salads. Quite simple and tasty salads can be made of such ingredients as cheese and sliced apple, or sardines and coleslaw. These can be carried to work in a plastic box and eaten without bread or other carbohydrate. They will be found quite satisfying if enough is taken.

Another adjustment that should cause little problem is to insist on having raw fruit as the sweet at the main meal in place of pudding or other sweet. Few landladies would object to this, particularly if the lodger bought his own fruit. She would be saved work.

Sugar in drinks can be given up altogether. The various substitutes on the market dramatically cut carbohydrate intake with no ill effect. Reducing the intake of bread and potatoes will complete the adjustment needed.

If you have read the earlier chapters of this book, you should have no difficulty in working out what steps are necessary and possible in your particular case.

As well as the problem of too many calories, however, people faced with a diet over which they do not have complete control may find that they are deficient in one or more of the essential nutrients. This deficiency will make itself felt in time. Their answer here must be to supplement their diet with extras. The following are the most commonly used supplements:

BREWER'S YEAST

This is sold in powdered form and is rich in the B vitamins and in minerals and amino acids. It is usually sprinkled on milk, water, tomato or fruit juice. It can also be mixed with water in the proportion of 2 tablespoonfuls to a pint to form a drink. People who do not like the natural taste can buy flavoured varieties. It can also be obtained straight from the brewery in thick liquid form rather like black treacle, and this whilst not quite as nice as golden syrup, is palatable and can be eaten by the spoonful.

COD-LIVER OIL

Most of us are familiar with this, since it is an old remedy and readily available at chemists. It supplements vitamin D. Since it also aids the absorption of calcium into our system it is especially good for brittle bones and hence for old people. Taken with citrus fruits and blackcurrants it helps to ward off winter colds.

WHEAT GERM

This is one of the best sources of vitamin E. It also contains iron and the B vitamins, and is very rich in protein. It is usually added to cereals but may be cooked in milk and eaten in this form as a cereal. Half a cup may be used as a part substitute for an equal quantity of flour in making cakes.

BRAN

Bran provides roughage, and we have spoken of its use in relieving constipation and promoting regularity of the bowel movements earlier in this book. It is to be found in health stores and looks rather like sawdust, but is quite palatable when sprinkled over other cereal or on soup, or when taken by the spoonful and washed down with a drink. I would recommend regular daily doses of this for health.

POWDERED SKIM MILK

Skim milk is simply milk with the butter fat removed. At one time no one would dream of drinking skim milk unless too poor to afford ordinary milk. On farms it was fed to pigs. For slimmers, however, skim milk is ideal, since it has one tenth of the fat content of ordinary milk and yet contains ten times the amount of protein. Skim milk is rich in calcium, protein, vitamin B_2 and other nutrients. It can be used to enrich ordinary milk by adding a tablespoonful to a pint, or it can be mixed with water and used instead of ordinary milk for cooking. It makes excellent rice puddings etc. The easiest way to buy and store it is in tins.

BLACK TREACLE

This contains the B vitamins, iron and calcium. It can be eaten on its own by the spoonful, spread on bread like golden syrup, stirred into milk or used as a substitute for sugar in any drink.

YOGHURT

This is a food well known to health food fans. It is a cultured milk product that is very easy to absorb in the digestive system where it manufactures the B vitamins. Yoghurt is rather an acquired taste and those who are not impressed with the natural flavour should try one of the fruit-flavoured forms first. Its food value is undoubted.

As well as adding food supplements to the diet, which may be necessary in some of the cases mentioned above, all readers will benefit from the aids to fitness suggested in the rest of this chapter.

SUNBATHING

The sun promotes the growth of all living things. When the weather permits, therefore, sunbathe as often as possible. Do not overdo it at first or your skin will burn. Try a few minutes a day until you start to acquire a tan, and if your skin is very sensitive use one of the protective oils. Gradually increase the time of exposure until you can spend as long as you like in the open air. Sunshine falling on the bare skin is a useful source of vitamin D.

SUN LAMPS

In winter or when there is an absence of sunshine, sunray lamps will be of similar value to sunshine itself. It is essential to follow any instructions that come with them, however, so as not to overexpose yourself. Some models are available on medical prescription only, and if you are using one of these you must follow your doctor's advice. The ones sold without prescription give exposure times. It is very little, being about one minute every four days in most cases. Do not on any account make the mistake of thinking they are the same as ordinary sunlight.

AIR BATHS

When it is not too cold, it is very helpful to expose the whole of your body to the air. The air not only tones up the skin but induces a feeling of relaxation and well-being. Your body is able to breathe freely through all its pores as well as through the nose. The benefits of nudism in its effect on one's whole attitude to life and in getting rid of tensions has been well known to naturists for years. You do not have to go as far as to join a nudist group; you can practise in privacy. Sleeping in the nude is also a wonderful tonic, and you will find that it promotes deeper and more natural rest with consequent benefit on your activities the next day.

COLD SHOWERS

Provided your heart is sound, a cold shower tones up the whole system and gives a glowing feeling of well-being. When you have a hot shower to cleanse yourself, turn the water to cold for the last minute or so. It will come as a shock at first but soon you will know the value.

TURKISH BATHS

An occasional Turkish bath opens all the pores in your body and thoroughly cleanses them. You will be amazed at how much hidden dirt comes out even though you wash frequently and well.

SAUNAS

The sauna is a Swedish way of achieving the same effect as Turkish baths. You lie in a pine-scented room heated by a charcoal brazier on which water is poured to create steam. In Sweden you beat yourself gently with twigs and this form of self-massage stimulates further perspiration and elimination of dirt.

MASSAGE

Massage tones up the muscles and leads to relaxation. You can perform simple self-massage with long strokes up the limb towards the heart and with circular movements, but full massage is best entrusted to experts, in whose hands it can be very beneficial in relieving strain or assisting healing.

Apart from all the diets, exercises and aids given in this book, however, fitness depends on one's attitude to life. A cheerful, optimistic, positive attitude goes a long way. A balanced life in which you devote a correct proportion of your time to work, to rest and to leisure will keep you on the right road. Try to strike a balance between physical and mental activities. If you work in an office all day, then seek recreations that take you out of doors or crafts that use your hands. If you are an outdoor worker, choose hobbies that stimulate the brain; read, listen to music, study something.

There is no need for people to feel that when they pass the age of thirty-five their sporting days are done. Many sports such as golf, swimming, cycling, badminton, judo and karate are practised by the old as well as young. Even when competitive days are over, walking is still a good way of getting exercise. Study your local evening-class programmes. They may give you new ideas as to physical or mental activities you could take up with benefit.

The ability to relax is important to health. It is the tense, nervous people who develop ulcers. Recent research in America indicates that meditation is valuable in improving our ability to cope with life. Whether you undertake serious transcendental meditation classes or simply make a quiet time for yourself each day, you will find it of help. Yoga is a study that assists relaxation also.

Seek the inward peace that will remain with you through any outward tribulation. Fitness concerns the whole man, and as well as being physical, is mental and spiritual in its dimensions.

Index